"Powerful, necessary, rejuvenating, and optimistic, this book delves into the ancient past as well as the emerging psychosocial field to explore 'mutual aid' as a proven archetypal social form oriented against oppressive hierarchy. Using the previously untold story of a successful mind-body response to the AIDS crisis, the authors joyfully demonstrate that mutual aid communities can be a decolonizing, empowering, psychodynamic, and artistic pathway to better lives."

Susan Rowland (PhD) teaches at Pacifica Graduate Institute and is author with Joel Weishaus of *Jungian Arts-based Research and the Nuclear Enchantment of New Mexico* (2021)

"*The Healing Power of Community* concretizes the authors' collective wisdom emerging from their shared dedication to empowerment and meaning-making through community suffering and solidarity. The spirit of their work during the AIDS crisis is enriched with theory, history, arts-based research, and practical guidance from psychodrama, mutual aid practices, liberation psychology, and Jungian analysis. An essential resource for anti-oppressive practitioners working with groups and communities."

Scott Giacomucci, DSW, LCSW, BCD, CGP, FAAETS, TEP, Director, Phoenix Center for Experiential Trauma Therapy; Author of *Social Work, Sociometry, & Psychodrama* (2021) and *Trauma-Informed Principles in Group Therapy, Psychodrama, & Organizations* (2023).

"*The Healing Power of Community* is not just an inspirational or informative resource, but a triumphant and urgent call for each of us to join together around our mutual concerns and to actively participate in the creation of a new consciousness!"

Nora Swan-Foster, Jungian Analyst, art therapist, former North American Editor of the *Journal of Analytical Psychology*, and author of *Jungian Art Therapy* and *Art Therapy and Childbearing Issues.*

"The connection of humanity contains our social suffering and facilitates transitions of collective darkness into the group healing process. This book not only demonstrates different ways of mutual aid for group healing but also bridges possible methods of applying psychodrama and depth psychology for improving social justice."

Siyat Ulon, MD, TEP Director of American Board of Examiners of Psychodrama, Sociometry and Group Psychotherapy.

T0383658

"The invincible courage to sustain a loving community in the time of AIDS is extraordinary. For me, it is deeply personal since I was working among healing physicians at San Francisco General Hospital in the 1980s. As these pandemics continue, it remains personal and this community's story of unshakable compassion is more important to share widely than ever."

Molly Osborne is an M.D., Ph.D., Professor of Medicine, OHSU, former OHSU Associate Dean of Student Affairs, Integrated Ethics Program Officer Portland VA Hospital

"The authors offer a remarkable integration of experience, psychology, and politics from the dark years of the AIDS crisis. It is rare to read records of groups from that time, and the authors offer powerful ways to bring their meanings forward into our present."

Paul Attinello, PhD, Jungian analyst, HIV/AIDS scholar

"The notion of humankind is marked by this book: Human Kind. It is the activity of human kind(ness) that must be realized now; if we are to survive. This book will offer a warm and kind, a caring and loving, a realistic and an optimistic path – a welcomed document long overdue and right on time."

Edward Schreiber, TEP, Director, Zerka Foundation, Amherst, MA

The Healing Power of Community

The Healing Power of Community offers a diverse cross section of interdisciplinary and depth-psychological perspectives in support of using mutual aid approaches in all levels of group and community practice as a remedy for individualism and social and political divisions, centering social justice.

Written by three distinct voices who collaborated at the height of the AIDS crisis, the book begins with an autoethnographic study of Project Quest, an HIV/AIDS clinic established in 1989, before looking at how the lessons learnt from this clinic can be applied to our current global mental health climate. Filled with clinical and theoretical applications, chapters include content on what mutual aid communities are, rethinking professionalism and boundaries in a crisis, healing collective trauma, group psychotherapy, psychodrama, depth psychology, and how mental health professionals can support radical change of key structures in nonprofit clinics, public administration, private practice, and research. Arguing for their approach of radicalizing mental health and community-based practice today, the book examines how this can be achieved by moving beyond individual-level approaches, creating new frameworks to meet the mental health needs of our era in creative ways.

This book is designed to engage clinical social workers and mental health care clinicians working in community-based mental health, as well as those involved in community psychology, collective trauma and grief, HIV/AIDS advocacy, policy making, and political advocacy.

Lusijah Marx is a nurse, clinical psychologist, and psychedelic facilitator in Portland, OR. She co-founded the Quest Center for Integrative Health Care, a wellness-based healthcare nonprofit, and founded Radiance Integrative Health and Wellness.

Graham Harriman is a long-term survivor of HIV, a psychotherapist, and Chair of the CAEAR Coalition. Most recently he also served as the Director of the HIV Health and Human Services Planning Council of New York at the NYC Department of Health and Mental Hygiene.

Robin McCoy Brooks is a Jungian analyst, nationally certified Trainer, Educator, and Practitioner of group psychotherapy, sociometry, and psychodrama, and author of *Psychoanalysis, Catastrophe & Social Change* (2022), winner of the "best book" award by the International Association for Jungian Studies.

The Healing Power of Community

Mutual Aid, AIDS, and Social Transformation in Psychology

Lusijah Marx, Graham Harriman, and Robin McCoy Brooks

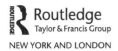
Routledge
Taylor & Francis Group

NEW YORK AND LONDON

Designed cover image: The cover art was painted by Roger Bell entitled "Killer Bees," donated to Project Quest in 1996. Roger used guided imagery of killer bees to keep himself from going blind from the cytomegalovirus in the early 1990s.

First published 2025
by Routledge
605 Third Avenue, New York, NY 10158

and by Routledge
4 Park Square, Milton Park, Abingdon, Oxon, OX14 4RN

Routledge is an imprint of the Taylor & Francis Group, an informa business

ISBN: 978-1-032-47874-6 (hbk)
ISBN: 978-1-032-47873-9 (pbk)
ISBN: 978-1-003-38633-9 (ebk)

DOI: 10.4324/9781003386339

Typeset in Times New Roman
by codeMantra

We dedicate this book to Project Quest, to our mentors in living and dying, who taught us so much about love, courage, showing up, and the necessity of community.

Contents

Acknowledgements

We want to thank our many communities for helping us write the book we envisioned seven years ago.

Big love to Johnny Olesen for writing the Foreword of this book, and for regularly meeting with us, becoming a soul partner in our book's unfolding.

We are very grateful for our formidable colleagues who honored our work with their endorsements just when we needed a booster shot in our final push to the summit. They inspire us and give us courage. They are Nora Swan-Foster, Scott Giacomucci, Susan Rowland, Siyat Ulon, Paul Attinello, Ed Schreiber, and Molly Osborne.

With great luck, Paul Attinello was one of our "blind" reviewers. Robin recognized his commentary style and then his name at the bottom of a page. His lengthy and pithy critique was invaluable and greatly shaped the direction of our book. A hearty thanks to the other blind reviewer, who remains anonymous, yet their input directed us to write a lengthy Part I section, more fully contextualizing the hidden history of mutual aid, including the luminaries of group and community psychology in the last century.

Thank you to Greg Fowler for sharing your private journal excerpts with us and enriching our efforts to recall the complexities of those early days of AIDS.

Big love for Dale Buchanan and John Mosher, who annually led Quest psychodrama men's retreats in the later AIDS era.

We want to thank the Routledge editorial team for their excellent support throughout.

We are indebted to and humbled by our colleagues, friends, and Quest community members with whom we shared many life-changing experiences that resulted in the creation of Project Quest, including co-founder Lucas Harris, Wasaka Borgelt, Jessie Isaac, Gregory Fowler, Robby Smith, Mary Kimsey, Bill Brooks, Molly Osborne, Jim O'Hearn, Dale Buchanan, John Mosher, Greg Carrigan, Tabor Porter, "Connie," Aaron Hornstein, Ken Ballard, Brice Winters, Casey Merideth, Deb Gruber, Jeffrey Burdick, Shellie Barich, Colleen Groll, Saskia Von Micholovski, Mar-Gilsen-Mendel, Michael Mickow, Romy Royce,

Lusana Hubbard, Monica Spooner, Travis Penn, John Wicher, Tad Williams, Paul Moore, Joy Halme, Dave Nimmons, Roger Bell, Brian Bonus, Jack Cox, Jeff Owens, Sydney Thompson, Bonnie Blackwolf, Ayodeji Otuyelu, Adewale Olowu, Johnny Olesen, Erin Carruth, Wendy Neal, David Eisen, Bess Pinon, Catherine Adler, Joseph Sprietsma, Christopher Carloss, Jack Leaven, Deb Gruber, Michelle Barich and Monica Spooner.

Lusijah: I want to thank Lucas Harris for his courage, unwavering faith, and sense of humor that allowed Project Quest to emerge. My gratitude to our first cohort of Questers, Brian Bounous, Roger Bell, Jack Cox, Micah Smith, Bob Harrington, Dan Pillars, Greg Carrigan, Luke Lyons, and David Berry, who taught me so much. I want to thank my beloved friends and courageous colleagues Graham and Robin, who helped form the foundation of Quest with our shared belief in community and mutual aid. They showed a willingness to work tirelessly to sustain Project Quest, and later to know that "we needed to write it down" and pass along and inspire others with our experience and what we learned. I have appreciation for Leo Marx, who supported me and Quest financially in the beginning, and for my children Robert, Lionel, Miriam, and Hilary, who always inspire and sustain me. I honor and love my sister Mary Kimsey, a key part of my community who gives me strength, along with Molly Osborne and Marius Harold. Thank you to David Eisen for his support in helping Quest thrive and become what it is today. I want to acknowledge Renata Ackermann, Wendy Neal, Wasaka Borgelt, and Gloria Nepstead as friends who helped build the Quest community. My Subud spiritual community deepened my belief in the Inner Intelligence/Inner Healer within each of us and I appreciate the members of that community who helped me believe in the necessity of acting with courage towards social justice and compassion and love for all beings. I have gratitude to Karen Hudes, who edited and helped and encouraged me as I wrote my chapters. I so appreciated her interest and belief in the value of this book.

Graham: I thank my great friend and previous partner Carlos Medina for his support through the most trying times of living with HIV. Without his unwavering support I would not be alive today. Of course, my family Katrina, Melinda, Rhys, and Ann, and Charles Harriman, Kelly Dennis, John Barry, and Bill Grennon have been amazing champions for me through my personal and professional challenges and successes. My husband Ayodeji Otuyelu, my sweetie Gian Carlos Flores, and Adewale Olowu provided continued feedback and support throughout the past several years that has been immeasurable. My colleagues at the New York City Department of Health provided much insight and experience that contributed to this book. For my writing process, I want to sincerely thank Karen Hudes for her tireless editing and feedback on each draft of each chapter. Dave Nimmons also provided excellent insight based on his decades of work as a gay psychologist working in the community.

Robin: Big love for my husband Ted Leonhardt and my extended family who inspired, challenged, and accompanied me, dead and alive, through the ordeals that background this book. They are Edna and Paul G. McCoy, Cheryl McCoy, Elliott Paul, and Amanda Brooks, and Bill Brooks who fully supported us in the Quest years and served on the Quest Board; AmySue, Eric, Bo, and Sam Leonhardt; and the social activist McCoy contingent – Barbi, Anne, and Paul McCoy.

I stand on the formidable shoulders of my mentors, Ladson Hinton, Leon Fine, Dale Buchanan, John Mosher, Jon Mills, Wolfgang Giegerich, Susan Rowland, Kevin Lu, Mark Saban, Paul Attinello, Rusty Palmer, and Gloria Anzaldúa. My psychodrama and Jungian roots mingle in the soil of this book.

I am very grateful for the creative and copy-editing efforts of Karen Hudes and Daniel Masler, who laboriously helped us shape each chapter.

A hearty thanks to Marianne Shapiro, who creatively edited Chapter 6.

All client material presented in this volume has been anonymized to protect identity and privacy.

Foreword

John Olesen

My heart was touched when Robin, Lusijah, and Graham asked me to write the Foreword for their book, *The Healing Power of Community: Mutual Aid, AIDS, and Social Transformation in Psychology.* Their reaching out pulled me back to the times we worked, cried, danced, and laughed together. Fear, isolation, confusion, and death marked this most virulent time of the AIDS epidemic. How were we to survive? Healing and creativity came from activists, artists, our friends, and the people living with AIDS themselves. Playing softball, climbing mountains, facing addictions, and delving into social phobias, or the spirals of spirituality, the Project Quest groups themselves were the conduits for the work of connecting and thriving. We all learned so much.

These authors changed me as a psychodramatist and as a therapist. More importantly, they incited me to question patriarchal authority and rules that served entrenched systems of power and dominance. They helped me pull back from the tendency to see everything as polarized, and therefore to categorize many others as enemies. They helped me to see that we are all in the maelstrom together. By leaning into each other, and into the depths of ourselves, we might survive and make our lives better. We can help one another.

I am one of the many who came of age during the dawn of gay liberation, only to watch entire circles of friends die of a mysterious illness as the government did nothing to help them. Living in New York City at that time, I had two circles of friends: gay men in 12-Step recovery rooms and men and women in the New York theater scene. In both groups, I watched my friends and mentors suffer. They endured physical torment from a ravaging disease and also suffered emotionally from cruel social ostracism, compounding the failure of the government and healthcare providers to honor their basic rights to obtain the medical care and other services that they needed so desperately. It was the plague, a time of cat-scratch fever, night sweats, and hazmat suits.

In the fall of 1983, despairing, I ventured outside my studio apartment to join other volunteers at the Gay Men's Health Center (GMHC), founded two years earlier by playwright Larry Kramer. As a volunteer, my assignment was to help out a person living with AIDS and attend small support groups, in people's apartments. Our small group managed to make us all feel safe about being vulnerable as our feelings of hopelessness and futility grew. Caring people and regular neighbors stepped forward to fill the void where institutions failed to address the concerns of people who were sick and fearful. Many asked, "How can I help?" They were willing to do whatever it took to provide for and comfort those in need.

I loved the city in the 1970s and early '80s. In those years, it was sexy, gritty, and naughty. Things felt deliciously illicit. Then, everything got scary—really scary. The dying became too much. Grief was beginning to swirl me. The small groups at GMHC couldn't support me enough. I needed to run, not walk, to the nearest exit.

I followed a boyfriend to Santa Fe, New Mexico. Still, AIDS was everywhere. In Santa Fe, I stumbled into working for New Mexico AIDS Services (NMAS). At NMAS, we were required to attend a two-weekend training with folks from California's Shanti Project, started by Dr. Charlie Garfield. Charlie's model of help equipped a volunteer caregiver with skills in listening, tolerance, and effective communication. Sometimes the work involved wielding a dust mop or delivering a sack of groceries for folks unable to get out. It gave me a focus, and a way to help.

Was I helping? How could I possible help more? Helping more required more knowledge and skill, so in 1989 I entered graduate school to study counseling psychology. While in school, I received a psychodrama internship with a nearly year-long commitment at Saint Elizabeth's Psychiatric Hospital in Washington, DC, far from the aspens and ponderosa pines of the Southwest. At Saint Elizabeth's, I learned that psychodrama is an experiential, action-based therapy that incorporates aspects of role playing, dramatic self-presentation, and group dynamics. Created by Jacob Moreno, a psychiatrist, and carried forward by his wife, Zerka Moreno, psychodrama has its own philosophy, methodology, and theory of human development. Additionally, it includes elements of theater and sociology.

Learning psychodrama was one thing, Saint Elizabeth's was another. There were tiny kids in the children's ward screaming at the monsters on the ceiling. In the adult wards, people rocked and whispered in corners. The forensic unit housed unrepentant rapists and pedophiles. Missing lightbulbs and basic supplies, the wards were dark, dirty, and smelled of urine—part of the dehumanizing system of the hospital itself. The feelings of hopelessness that I had known in New York were alive again.

Participating in the psychodrama program offered some relief. During my internship I watched my mentors greet the anguished people inside these wards with something rare in this setting—respect. I learned from them as they showed up and listened with their full attention. They seemed to lean into this other-worldly horror show with the deepest and most thoughtful positive regard.

Returning to Santa Fe wasn't easy for me. My job changed, and my boyfriend left. A friend in Seattle told me that there was an affordable apartment opening in his building, so I jumped at the chance to leave the relentless desert sun and sadness of a relationship that had ended and trade all of that for the cool, rainy weather of the Pacific Northwest.

Alone in Seattle, I researched how I might continue my psychodrama studies. I met Robin McCoy Brooks, a Trainer, Educator, and Practitioner (TEP) of psychodrama. I found her to be warm, brilliant, and, a bit mysteriously, shy about her work. I could tell that she was glad to meet me. She knew about St. Elizabeth's Hospital and my training, and she was curious about my AIDS work.

Robin told me about Project Quest co-founded by Lusijah Marx. She invited me to meet Lusijah and Graham Harriman, a young psychotherapist, and attend a Project Quest retreat. I expressed my concerns about perhaps not fitting in because I was HIV-negative. How could I possibly help? She gently pointed out that she was also HIV-negative and not gay. We had a laugh. It was an *Oh, hell yes. I know that feeling!* kind of laugh, a connection of a deeper knowing. I remember that Robin said the group would either accept me, or not accept me, but this would probably not be based on my HIV status. Then she looked at me for a moment. Here was that unconditional positive regard I learned about in Washington, DC, being refocused onto me.

Nonetheless, I was still nervous about my first Quest retreat. I knew that it was going to be different from other retreats that I had attended. The physical space was tight. I found myself sleeping on the floor with other retreat participants. The APA guidelines flashed in my mind. Where were the clear boundaries between leaders and participants? Was this why Robin was mysterious? Were they all friends? Was being friends allowed? My role was unclear. Staff, participant, observer? I was none of these roles. I was each. While my role seemed confusing, the casual acceptance from everyone in the group was not. I had entered a community. People were curious about what I was doing there, but even more curious about who I was. I was accepted and respected just for showing up. My first night, I relaxed and exhaled among the sweetness of the snores and other sounds of men. The rigid boundaries I had learned between client and therapist seemed far away and irrelevant. Where would we go?

I remember watching Robin direct a psychodrama the next day. A very frail younger man put himself forward to do some "unfinished business." Hollow-eyed, he was small and fragile. Whatever he needed from Robin, or the group, it had to be gentle. Robin's care came through in her presence. She opened herself and listened to him. She asked him about his "unfinished business." With a raspy voice, he stated quietly that he might never know what it was to have a loving partner, and that he was very sad. I looked around the room and sensed the consensus from the group that he was probably correct. Severely ill, he was long past the time for dating, or romance. Still, his yearning remained strong. Practical and focused, Robin helped him unpack what he wanted from a lover:

just someone to hold him and love him. He wanted someone to eat popcorn with while watching movies in bed.

I felt my own wave of grief. Robin didn't sugarcoat his situation, offer platitudes, or suggest paths to acceptance. Instead, she gave him the opportunity to claim, weak as he was, what he wanted through psychodrama. Getting his permission to explore, she turned to the group and asked if there was anyone who would be willing to play his lover. Quietly, hands were raised around the room. These were loving hands from everyone—absolutely everyone—in the room. The willingness felt like a hum.

Robin guided us in a delicate dance of a ritual where the guys in the group would take turns playing his would-be lover, climbing into an imaginary bed made of chairs and blankets and gently holding him. Not one of these auxiliary ego actors needed any role training or needed to be shown how to be. I remember how quiet it was as we fell under the spell of our shared collective reality. Lovers' giggles and secret whispers joined the inevitable awkwardness about getting the pillows and physical entanglements of ailing bodies just right. There was an abundance of time, yet each of us felt the evaporating preciousness of each lover, each moment, each breath. When he felt complete, our protagonist sat up in the bed by himself. He looked to Robin and the group and simply said, "Yes, that is what I wanted. That is what I needed. Thank you."

Usually, at the end of each drama, there is a sharing in which the audience members and people who played auxiliary roles express to the protagonist how the drama affected them personally. The sharing from this group was minimal, yet powerful. People simply stated that they would be honored to have him as a lover. We all could be lovers for each one of us.

In psychodrama, the Here and Now dominates. Dramas about past events are played in the present. The same is true for dramas that explore the future. Watching this drama unfold, I discovered that in struggling to be alive and to live fully, each of us can become our own next chance, perhaps our last chance, to be welcomed, understood, and accepted.

Through example and through a sometimes clunky improvisational dance of creativity, Robin, Lusijah, and Graham introduced me to a new way of using my full self and a deeper knowing to be with others. I took the three of them with me in my mind and heart when I moved to California and worked for the Shanti Program. How were they staying present and navigating nonprofit agency frustrations, the complexities and politics of public administration, and the isolation and puzzles inherent in private practice? I experienced my own outrage at the maddening, overall direction of healthcare corporatization. At the same time, this rage didn't overpower me. Thankfully, Robin, Lusijah, and Graham taught me to connect with a deeper sense of what is in the moment, based on the souls in the room, the messages from our own human bodies, and the insight of those who came before us. They continue to help me remember to allow space for not knowing and to hold the possibility of truth and healing beyond my limited scope. Their strength helps me trust the moment just before spontaneity transforms that which was into something new.

When Graham, now at the New York State Department of Public Health, invited Shanti to come to New York City and share a holistic model of health I knew that these values could travel from heart to heart across distance and twisted obstacles. Our sociometric circles could intersect, each helping the other.

I believe our collective work is rooted in what Zerka Moreno called tele, a mutual connection and communication of deep knowing. It is surely a place of open regard and respect in which the student teaches the teacher, and vice versa. Just as the auxiliaries knew instinctively how to play loving partners, I believe there is a chance we all will know the "next right thing" if we allow ourselves to be present, connected, authentic, and vulnerable.

There are all kinds of pockets of inequity, cruelty, and suffering. Mutual aid, recovery, and resilience require us to challenge the structures of power and the ways we've worked in the past. Any challenge is sure to find pushback. In this moment, we are polarized by many factors, emotionally, politically, and culturally. The radical stance that Graham, Robin, and Lusijah put forward requires change. As we all know, change, whatever form it takes, can be painful.

Once I asked a group of men and women living with AIDS where they went when there was too much pain. Each person in our group had a particular place he or she had discovered. These were the corners of respite while having a tooth drilled, a catheter inserted, or receiving devasting news. After sharing all of these special magical places, we, as a group, chose one to enact as a psychodrama.

Our chosen place was offered by a divorced mom with three kids. She was a regular Project Quest retreat participant and a client of the day program at Seattle's Bailey-Boushay House, the AIDS hospice where I worked. Susan (not her real name) adjusted her IV pole and took us through the magic of surplus reality to her green hill, overlooking a pond at the edge of an apple orchard where all the apple trees were in blossom.

We all were with her as caring friends, fellow sufferers, and little ducks under her motherly wings. We were caretakers of her and of one another. We all dared to follow her. We smiled as the warm breeze stirred the apple blossoms around us. We wore white summer clothes and felt free. Someone from the group noticed a beautiful old tree with a strong trunk and arching branches. Holding hands, we each lay at its soft grassy base and looked at the bluest of blue skies through the leaves. Breathing together we were safe. It seemed so perfect.

Suddenly, I felt panic set in. How could we ever leave? How could we return to her green garden hill? As we sat up, the group shot me a frightened look that I was souring the drama and thrusting us all back to an unbearable world.

Susan smiled and took my hands. She told me that we could all return to the tree and sky and apple blossoms simply by imagining her face and entering into her eyes. Susan, with her motherly wisdom, assured us that going through the portals to new places doesn't have to be complicated or difficult. Our group relaxed. We spent a bit of time practicing looking into her eyes, and each other's eyes. Our group knew she was right.

This mutual aid intimacy work can hurt and the landscape is gnarly. We need places of respite because they are essential to confront the current care systems and the paradigms that we have in place that determine who gets helped, and the forms and timetables for what help is available. There has to be a better way, one that is more respectful of people and their needs. With an incoming tide, all boats rise. In our humanness, there is abundance. As Thich Nhat Hanh said, "the next Buddha will be a Sangha."* We need to look into each other's eyes.

How can I help? Perhaps that is not quite the best question. How can *we* help and accept help ourselves? Like many, I have the natural inclination to compartmentalize. Oh, that was the time of the AIDS Crisis. That was the Covid time. Robin, Lusijah, and Graham have decompartmentalized and pulled essential learning from deep pain. I encourage you to read and feel into the lived experience and wisdom of this book. I encourage you to be open to the possibility of real transformation for yourself, and for all of us. Together we can do what I cannot do alone.

---

* A sangha is a Buddhist religious community or monastic order.

Introduction

*Robin McCoy Brooks, Graham Harriman,
and Lusijah Marx*

Millennial Mutual Aid

Mutual aid surfaces in the timeless stories of living with people and facing life in dangerous times. Scholarly studies of mutual aid groups, movements, and societies show us how egalitarian networks are the incubators of democratic community from which the freedom to create different forms of social reality becomes possible (Hartman, 2021).[1] In contrast, the forces of capitalism and colonialism have resulted in fundamentally un-democratic systemic structures in politics, business, and healthcare. Social groups based on profit, exploitation, and empire are controlled by a small percentage of people who determine our fates, numb our abilities to relate meaningfully to each other, and repress new liberatory realities.[2] Rigid hierarchical social structures that valorize rugged individualism and competition for resources alienate us from the memory of how we have connected to each other through the ages (Spade, 2020; Wright, 2014).

There are more optimistic and hopeful accounts in the history of civilization, however, that have startling implications for how we can imagine new forms of organizing society at the most fundamental level, beginning in our own house. Anthropologist David Graeber and archaeologist David Wengrow refute the idea that centralized government, through layers of hierarchical bureaucracy, is the only rational or workable political system to govern the masses.[3] Peoples across the globe, they reason, have historically been making conscious, deliberate, collective, and creative choices about how they organized their societies, apportioned wealth and work, distributed power, and practiced politics without the need of centralized control or administration. In their study of 200,000 years of human history they were able to find no evidence that supports the notion that war or other theaters of violence such as mass enslavement and prison camps, torture, and genocide have *always* existed (Graeber & Wengrow, 2021, pp. 505–524). Instead, their research offers evidence of intermittent occurrences of extreme warfare with alternating long periods of peace often lasting for centuries even, or millennia.

DOI: 10.4324/9781003386339-1

Archeological evidence from highly populated mega-sites (cities) supports their claims that mutual aid practices have been widely evidenced in the last 30,000 years of human history. They reference a number of largely populated city sites that indicate social organization without centralized administration, rank, and wealth distinctions (Ibid., pp. 284–358).[4] While richly varied, the economies of these cities often presented complex and logistical challenges (including managing ecosystems) that were resolved through intricate *fluid systems of collaboration* without any need for centralized or violent control (Ibid., pp. 294–297). Why, they wonder, do we remain fixed and seemingly unable to draw on the creative resources of our ancient ancestors, who for thousands of years invented and experimented with every imaginable form of social organization while consistently pursuing freedom, mutuality, and principally new knowledge systems? (Ibid., p. 519).

From a related perspective, evolutionary sociologist Nicholas Christakis cogently argues that all human beings share genetically "wired" social sensibilities that enable us to build "good societies." We are primed, he argues, for banding together, making friends, showing kindness, recognizing uniqueness, expressing reciprocal love, teaching what we know, learning socially, sharing resources, cooperation, and preferring mild hierarchy (Christakis, 2019, pp. 12–18). These social sensibilities are called upon when we pull together with all of our limitations, abilities, *and* differences to collectively act, as a form of civic responsibility, towards the creation of more liberatory social systems.

Most recently, mutual aid has gained broader recognition with the proliferation of widespread practice during the COVID-19 pandemic, as a way for communities to immediately share resources when governmental and other structures failed. Care was mobilized through the deeply ordinary labor of mutual relating from the knowledge that human life is beautiful, even in its most unglamourous or challenging times. This position is supported by the work of cultural critic Rebecca Solnit, who investigated in a 2009 publication a number of catastrophic disasters that took place in the last century. Her study reveals how the phenomena of mutual aid, altruism, and personal sacrifice, on behalf of others, blossoms in response to natural or human-engineered disasters. Think of a field of dandelions suddenly blooming under the right conditions.

Contemporary American scholars are re-envisioning history by drawing on many overlapping mutual aid informed revolutionary traditions that are negated by the accounts of history founded on Euro-white American exceptionalism (Anzaldúa, 1987; Nembhard, 2014; Pycior, 2014; Jones, 2020; Steele, 2020). Historian Chris Wright (2014) notes the accelerated tension that arose between the democratic, anti-authoritarian impulses of those who were drawn to mutual aid principles and the prevailing tendency of economic power structures to concentrate on ever-larger, more centralized, xenophobic, and coercive practices. Amidst this tension, we find a rich history of cooperation and communalism in the struggle for human rights. This is a different story than one of rugged individualism, unchecked capitalism, and colonializing oppression. We draw on these inclusive accounts of history to untangle how methods of social activism and resistance to oppression are linked to mutual aid practices in the history of the United States in Part I of this book.

Mutual Aid Meets Mental Health in the Vortex of AIDS

Our interest in mutual aid was heightened in our shared experiences over 30 years ago participating in the founding of a mutual aid, and mental health community during the onset of the AIDS crisis. From this community, a nonprofit clinic would be formed in 1989, named Project Quest.[5]

The Quest story began in the 1980s in Portland, Oregon, with Lusijah Marx's decision to design a psychoneuroimmunological protocol in her dissertation study. She would integrate key aspects of Eriksonian hypnotic guided imagery with the idea that the individual could improve their immune system's response against the encroaching HIV virus. As people increasingly joined her study, she quickly realized how rigorously the disease penetrated all aspects of their lives.

Receiving an AIDS diagnosis back then was a terrifying death sentence, and the death rate was surreal. Long-term survivor (LTS) Tabor Porter describes the "general malaise" of these early years as consuming: "Everybody was dying," and he was constantly afraid he would be next, or someone he knew and loved would be (Brooks, 2023, p. 48). Many people in Porter's life would delay being tested or did not talk about their status at all. "I would see somebody on the street one day, and then they would just disappear" (Ibid., p. 49). Porter experienced an omnipresent sense of dread, fear, isolation, and grief, along with feeling guilty for still being alive.

Greg Carrigan (LTS) describes his experience of those days as vacillating between the "unbearable intensity of not knowing if I would survive," juxtaposed with the unexpected ecstasy of "seeing a beautiful sky," and breaking into "uncontrollable weeping because I *was still alive*." "Remembering those times now are like a burning scar," he poignantly adds (Brooks, 2023, pp. 48–49).

When Lusijah first began her work in guided imagery with people with HIV and AIDS, she became quickly aware that there was a lack of infrastructure in the city to medically or psychologically care for those who were ill. Today, we have become accustomed to situations like this, where a government denies the far-reaching significance of a disaster, or abandons the afflicted, leaving them to deal with the horrific realities on their own. Or the government responds inadequately and/or distributes false news accounts about what is really happening on the ground. There is no viable choice then if we are dependent on systems that are inadequate and out of our control. Mutual aid projects allow us to relearn new, emancipatory ways of cultivating the practices and structures that mobilize us towards a shared goal, where each of us has a say in all parts of our lives.

In the 1980s, a zeitgeist of broader AIDS activism across the U.S. (and elsewhere) focused on the importance of empowering people living with HIV/AIDS.[6]

Restoring our humanity arose in the form of supporting each other by having each other's backs, sharing resources and information, coming together in coalitions to advocate for improvements (such as the FDA approval process), creating systems based on intergroup coordination that supported action, making our own treatment decisions, and challenging the top-down doctor/patient paradigm, to name only a few examples. Seeking health was born from a desire to survive in a culture that left us on the margins, to fight for ourselves. And fight for ourselves, with and among our allies, we did (Denver Principles, 1983; Halkitis, 2015; France, 2016; Schulman, 2021).

From these surrounds, Lusijah knew she needed to expand her therapeutic frame to include working in groups. She needed to secure a regular gathering place where meaningful connections with others could be made within a community because so many individuals were isolated, sick, and dying alone. She recruited allies within her immediate professional world, one at a time. She asked Robin McCoy Brooks, with whom she had previously trained and worked alongside in other contexts, to help her lead psychodrama retreats. Psychodrama is a comprehensive form of action-based, group psychotherapy that is mutual aid and social justice oriented.

Simultaneously, Graham Harriman, as a newly credentialed young gay therapist, asked to be a part of the forming community. Each of us had psychodrama training and a depth psychology orientation in common. Graham's desire to make a difference before he died (he thought then) uniquely contributed to the plurality of efforts that gave birth to the Quest community. Graham's position was unique because he was a gay man living with HIV disease, and a therapist. He knew many of the community members personally, and was challenged to break new therapeutic ground because of the dual roles he engaged in.

The vision of forming the mind/body clinic named Project Quest would come to Lusijah and Lucas Harris—an early collaborator—during one of our early psychodrama retreats. Lucas was one of the first participants in Lusijah's original study. On the same night, both Lucas and Lusijah had a dream of starting an AIDS healing center together. Years later, Lucas would die of AIDS in the spring of 1996, the same year a newly developed class of antiretrovirals (HAART) became a treatment option.[7] Lusijah would continue to work in the nonprofit clinic she co-founded to the present day. Project Quest is now named the Quest Center for Integrative Health.

How We Came to Write This Book: Graham's Vision of Returning to the Well

After the antivirals (HAART) became available in the late 90s, the height of the AIDS crisis began to wane into the 21st century. Each of us dispersed, developing separate career paths. Graham moved to New York City, taking a public health position in HIV care and program administration. He directed public policy, planning and HIV advocacy. Presently, he is a practicing psychotherapist and public health consultant.

In 2016, Graham and Robin were sitting on a park bench outside of Robin's Seattle office. Graham was attending a conference in Seattle, so they grabbed an hour before he needed to catch a cab to the airport. After catching up with key life events, the conversation fell into a pregnant lull. Graham's whole body suddenly filled with animated intensity. "*Why didn't we write it down?*" he suddenly blurted. We had been ignoring a shared part of our history.

Within seconds we were both crying from the emotional release of flooding memories that had deeply tethered the three of our lives. Graham's soul explosion was generated from the yearning to "return to the well," as he stated it then. He wanted to return to the vital edge of the work that emphasized the empowerment of person and group within their environment, the centrality of relationships and social justice. In healing spaces such as these, many dimensions of meaning-making possibility may awaken us to a concrete purpose that has not yet been realized in ourselves or in the world. The Quest community was such a place—where the aspirations of many individuals were materialized, and supported, often furthering a collective purpose in the maw of AIDS.

Within the week, we met with Lusijah. Graham's question ripped through each of us and opened us to the visceral memory of AIDS, reminding us how our collaborative relationship as therapists had irrevocably altered the course of our lives, and would again in the process of writing this book. The question became the portal through which we would each wrestle with memories containing both horrific intensity and the transformative power the Quest community had. We wrote *The Healing Power of Community* as we had worked together then, through a slow and arduous creative process of exhilarating, and painful, recollection, reflection, trial, error, and discovery.

We consider our book to be an arts-based research (ABR) project (Leavy, 2018). Jungian scholar Susan Rowland describes Jungian arts-based research (JABR) as a qualitative paradigm that "makes the mind and body of the researcher the chief organ of knowledge-gathering and knowledge-making" (Rowland, 2023, p. 437). As such, we co-engage quantitative and qualitative research design with personal experience, self-reflection, and imagination to generate new meanings for our present era. Our reflections are at times personally intimate. Our intimacy with each other pulls us into our depths and back out again into the various areas of concern, interest, and urgency that we write about together, and alone.[8]

Mutual Aid in the Field of Psychology

Our collaborative approach in working with groups, we later discovered, has remarkable similarities to how social activist Dean Spade (2020) describes group processes within activist mutual aid communities, described further in Part I.

Mutual aid communities are participatory and collectively solve problems without waiting for the help of dysfunctional social and governmental systems. Such cultures distribute power (leadership) so that issues/goals are collectively identified and addressed. Community members are thus mobilized toward shared aims, generated from the grassroots, versus a top-down, hierarchical power dynamic.

We found that the residential therapy retreats greatly contributed to the formation of what became a *hybrid mental health and mutual aid community*, on several counts.[9] First, Quest tended to the survival needs of those who were ill and disenfranchised from society. Attending to their psychological needs, within various modes of therapy, also allowed group members to share their individual experiences of the disease, as well as build a social network that shared emerging treatments.

Second, mutual aid communities are participatory in that they collectively solve problems without waiting for help from a dysfunctional social system or government (Spade, 2020, p. 16). [10] Third, mutual aid communities build a kind of solidarity that is essential to mobilizing the many towards shared aims, especially in a societal vacuum that blatantly disregards sites of injustice (p. 12). In our mutual aid–oriented psychodrama therapy groups, we found that social cooperation was linked to social bonding. Mutual aid communities become a facilitating mechanism for group cohesion. Group cohesion is furthered still by both a desire to survive and a chaotic urge to live fully that lies at the root of personal and collective agency.

Many of us have *not* been in groups whose processes are transparent, fair, and participatory, and where everyone is encouraged to participate in decision making. In mainstream psychology, we are usually not trained to notice or care about how our various groups are functioning, nor do we have a means of evaluating a group's dynamics. Much of the material in textbooks, academic journals, popular works of fiction, and nonfiction reflect the attitudes and biases that shape Euro-Western cultural psychology, with little acknowledgment of the value of group therapy. It may seem difficult to imagine we have the capacity to create intricate, fluid systems of mutual aid by opening up to a multi-versal framework that learns from a culturally rich foundation.

A Turn to Psychosocial Studies

The field of psychology is a vast archipelago including many diverse disciplines. While many traditions have begun to incorporate multiculturalism into their conversations, there remains considerable concern about how we can actually integrate the lived experience of those who are on the margins within our profession and communities at large.[11]

Within the last two decades, a new approach to social and psychological research has slowly emerged, termed "*psychosocial studies*" (Frosh, 2003). Contemporary psychosocial studies perceive the individual as both social and psychological, and as such constituted by many social formations. There are several developing tributaries that we draw on in this book, referred to as *applied psychoanalysis*. This is a term used to describe how psychosocial theorists have extrapolated aspects of depth psychology to explore unconscious processes in group and community relations, institutions, cultures, and historical eras (Hook, 2008; Wu, 2013; Frosh, 2015; Saban, 2020; Layton, 2023).

A few, but increasingly more psychoanalytic, writers and clinicians are addressing how socially shaped unconscious processes emerge in analysis *and are clinically worked with* (Brooks, 2023; Layton, 2023). Layton describes this emerging variation as *"clinical social psychoanalysis"* or *"psychosocial psychoanalysis"* (Layton, 2023). The origins of this mode of psychosocial studies are derived from depth psychology, applied social studies, social work, critical social psychology, social constructionism, queer theory, psychoanalytic feminist theorists, feminist social research, critical race theory, and liberation psychology (Frosh & Baraitser, 2008; Layton, 2023).

Psychosocial psychoanalytic studies draw on the works of Eric Fromm, Franz Fanon, Ignacio Martín-Baró, Kimberlé Crenshaw, Gloria Anzaldúa, Jessica Benjamin, Michael Foucault, Jacques Lacan, Judith Butler, and Slavoj Žižek, to name a few. It must be noted that while the founder of liberation psychology, Ignacio Martín-Baró, is happily included in this list, other luminaries of group and community research and practice are not, including J. L. Moreno and William Schwartz who, among other social workers, introduced the concept of "mutual aid" into the field of group social work in the 1960s.

Our book is a contribution to the fields of psychosocial studies, applied depth psychology, and psychosocial depth psychology. Part II of our book describes the penetrating effects of receiving an HIV-positive diagnosis in the personal and social spheres. We discuss the unconscious and conscious connections between the psyche and the social by exploring the interplay between individual and group processes, institutions, cultures, and historical contexts. Our book focuses on the application of liberatory and mutual aid–based approaches in group and community work as *a psychological remedy* to our culture's retreat into individualism, societal breakdown of community, and collective loss of *Eros*.[12] The larger questions about the kinds of societies that are possible in liberatory community and group processes is an over-arching theme.

We draw on depth psychology, especially Jungian and relational psychoanalysis.[13] We integrate elements of and mutual aid approaches to group and community practice, especially psychodrama (and sociodrama), and liberation psychology, a field of inquiry that is largely missing in psychosocial research (Giacomucci, 2021; Ordóñez, 2021; Layton, 2023). Only in 2018, for example, did the American Psychological Association recognize group psychology and group psychotherapy as a specialty practice (Whittingham et al., 2021).

Our intellectual ancestors in group and community psychology are Jacob Levy Moreno, the originator of the term group psychotherapy and the founder of psychodrama, sociometry, and sociodrama, referenced above, Ignacio Martín-Baró, and William Schwartz (Moreno, 1953; Schwartz, 1959; Martín-Baró, 1994). Psychodrama, liberation psychology, and social worker group epistemologies and practices overlap in their emphasis on egalitarianism and mutual aid, placing social justice at the center of training, practice, and research.

Healing and transformation through self-knowledge is possible in the context of group, community development and socio-political action. Another shared basic assumption is that the psychological dynamics of the individual are inseparable from the socio/political/eco realm. Thus, the liberation of the individual and their social and ecological milieu is inextricably tied to the transformation of society.

Following a liberatory approach means we must examine and amend the ways in which our theories and practices are bound to North American and Western Euro-centric perspectives that define healing from a universal frame. Intersectionality theory and practice move beyond a single-axis perspective to include a more nuanced understanding of the ways in which intersecting systems of oppression uniquely marginalize individuals in society and groups (Crenshaw, 1989). Intersectional theory was beginning to surface in the late 1980s through the scholarship of Black and other feminists of color who challenged the impact of unchecked institutional and structural oppression on individuals and communities from legal, historical, philosophical, and psychological perspectives (Anzaldúa, 1987; Hooks, 2014; Jones, 2020; Steele, 2020).

Contemporary psychology scholars continue to challenge the master grammar that defines healing from a universal frame versus a *differential* frame (Comas-Diaz, 2007; French et al., 2020). New health-promoting practices are being advanced, along with more discerning understandings about marginalization at the intersection of race, sexual identity, gender, neuro and bio-diversities, emigration status, and class oppression. These conceptual foundations for healing are grounded in cultural authenticity, collectivism, strength and resistance, and self-knowledge (Dykstra, 2014; Hancock 2016; Gill-Peterson, 2018; Belkin & White, 2020; Ordóñez, 2021).

Let us give an example of how we inadvertently retained a *universal-axis* (one psychology fits all) framework versus a differential (multi-versal) framework, which contributed to the further marginalization of people of color and Indigenous individual group members in the Quest community. As co-leaders, we had the privileges that came with being white, educated, and upper middle class. Lusijah and Robin were women therapists in a predominantly (but not exclusively) gay community. Graham was not an outsider, as a gay man living with HIV. The experience of living with HIV disease, for a white, well-educated gay man, however, comes with privileges and access to resources that many people in the Quest community did not share. Graham discusses this dynamic in Chapters 5 and 8.

One way we assumed a universal frame was through our subtle conflation of these distinctions and over-focusing on what group members had in common, in this case the experience of living with HIV disease. From our perspective, it is desirable to work with the "group as a whole," in an effort to track and explore emerging shared human themes to build group cohesion. However, we disregarded how the intersecting systems of oppression (gender, race, class, culture) *uniquely marginalized* the experience of living with AIDS.

Perhaps more people of color with an HIV-positive diagnosis, in the Portland area, would have considered participating in Quest if we had worked from a broader differential focus. A more inclusive space could have provided richer, deeper sharing of cultural heritage, rituals, and traditions that speak to the core of who one is (Watkins, 2019; French et al., 2020; Ruiz, 2020).[14] The process of self-critique is painful. Accepting accountability for the harm we inflicted because of our opacity, and facing our shame and guilt, continues to be an important part of our process, analysis, change, and message. In the words of Paulo Freire: "Those who undergo it [a liberatory path] must take on a new form of existence: they cannot any longer remain as they were" (Freire, 1994, p. 61).

Probably many of us practicing in healthcare and psychology today value the basic principles of democratic process, egalitarianism, and social justice. We hope that our volume's unfolding purpose will inspire our readers to put these values into action and push the boundaries of our field by placing mutual aid approaches at the very center of our clinical practice, advocacy, training, and research. We believe that there is a slow revolutionary turn towards community and group practice, whose embers we would like to enflame.

Presentation of Chapters

The Healing Power of Community is organized in three parts. In the broadest of brush strokes, Part I, entitled "Scientific, Activist, Historical, and Psychological Roots of Mutual Aid," describes mutual aid from multiple perspectives, organized into three chapters. Our intention is to orient the reader to a broad historical legacy of mutual aid that we later extend into group and community psychology today.

Chapter 1 explores the evolutionary roots of the term mutual aid, followed by contemporary research that supports our genetic and sociological capacities to form liberatory societies. The reader is oriented to basic components of mutual aid within survival activist cultures, illustrated by the Common Ground Relief project formed to support residents of Hurricane Katrina in New Orleans in 2005. The relationship between resilience and mutual aid is defined and elaborated.

Chapter 2 contains a survey of the hidden history of mutual aid movements within marginalized communities that arose prior to and after the last century in the United States. We draw on contemporary scholars who adopt an inclusive movement approach to re-envision an American history that draws on the many overlapping revolutionary traditions that actively challenge pervasive ideologies founded on Euro-white American exceptionalism and racial capitalism. Just as mutual aid remains a vital force within the invisibilized communities of American society today, so has it quietly resided in the background of community and group psychology in the last century.

Chapter 3 explores three visionaries of group and community psychology in the last century who were social justice and mutual aid oriented. These luminaries are Jacob Levy Moreno, Ignacio Martín-Baró, and William Schwartz.

Part II, entitled "The Quest Story," explores the conditions that contributed to the formation of an AIDS community that produced an AIDS clinic named Project Quest in 1989. We adopt an autoethnographic approach to explore our critically held personal experiences in relation to and with the experiences of others who were there. We survey the unique struggles of many individuals within a process of figuring out what to do, how to live, and how to make meaning of an existence that has suddenly lost its foundation amidst a crisis (Adams et al., 2015). Additionally, we rely on letters, pictures, newspaper accounts, artifacts, videos, poetry and other works of art, and historical accounts by other authors from different parts of the United States.

In Chapter 4, Lusijah Marx, co-founder of Project Quest, describes how a nonprofit AIDS clinic was formed from the energies of a vital mutual aid community in 1989. The vision for an AIDS clinic emerged from a shared nighttime dream that Lusijah and Lucas Harris received during an AIDS psychodrama retreat. This chapter tells the story of how this unique organization was co-created by the many efforts of a compassionate community. Quest provided a place where people became empowered by supporting each other and advocating for what they needed. It is also Lusijah's personal growth story among others who were involved in shaping Quest's unfolding purpose.

In Chapter 5, Graham Harriman relates his experience as a psychotherapist living with AIDS in the pre-antiretroviral treatment (ART) era. This role required a redefinition of professional boundaries to be able to develop effective therapeutic relationships and empathy to meet the needs of a community in crisis. He describes the importance of the dual-role relationship in a mutual aid community therapeutic model. The challenges of managing self-care in the midst of shared experiences between therapist and client are elaborated. Graham illustrates his narrative with the clinical challenges he encountered leading a sex addiction group attended by friends, and describes how he developed new methodologies in the treatment of sex addiction that were humane and non-shaming.

In Chapter 6, Robin McCoy Brooks discusses the efficacy of using a mutual aid approach to group therapy and community building within the context of a crisis situation. Drawing on journal excerpts from a Quest participant, she examines the existential and physical concerns that commonly emerged in the early era of AIDS. The basic principles of psychodrama theory and practice are described and illustrated. Robin follows the development of the group process in a single AIDS retreat that began with a horrific event. This event would facilitate the emergence of a collective theme about a shared desire to form meaningful friendship. This theme was explored and programs were developed beyond the retreat based on participant input. The inevitability of engaging in dual-role relationships among therapists and participants is also explored.

Part III is entitled "Re-visioning the Nonprofit Clinic, Public Program Administration, and Depth Psychology in Mental Health Today." It extracts key aspects of what we learned from building a hybrid mental health and mutual aid culture during the AIDS crisis and applies it towards re-envisioning psychology today. We integrate elements of liberation psychology, group and community practice, intersectionality theory, psychosocial theory, arts-based research, and depth psychology. Each of us contributes a chapter from our distinct career position today, offering concrete, practical, and innovative suggestions.

In Chapter 7, Lusijah Marx reflects on the evolution of the Quest Center for Integrative Health, with its grassroots beginnings remaining at its core. With Quest's growth, compromises came with receiving government funding. Lusijah faced the limitations of her shifting role, and questioned how the rules impact the people who need services most. She launched a new mutual aid initiative— branching off to a new path.

In Chapter 8, Graham Harriman describes how the politics of Quest over three decades ago relates to the need for raising and centering community voice in public health and mental health program administration for effective change. This includes broadening our definition of public health and mental health through an approach that starts with social determinants of health (poverty, income, race, class, neighborhood, education, etc.) and the incorporation of prevention and wellness, as well as recognition of the mind/body connection. He advocates for use of a holistic approach for integrated health and mental health through the combined effort of consumers, paraprofessionals, navigators, professionals, and program administrators.

In Chapter 9, Robin McCoy Brooks describes C. G. Jung's method of active imagination as a conduit for contemporary application. She elaborates on the writing practices of Gloria Anzaldúa, who used active imagination as a vehicle for activist arts-based research (ABR). Susan Rowland's creation of a new category of ABR, termed Jungian arts-based research, is discussed. Robin describes and illustrates her approach using Moreno's basic principles (tele, group cohesion, co-unconscious) of mutual aid group practice *with* aspects of Jung's method of active imagination (archetypes as themes, amplification). In this way, she extends Jung's methodology into concrete collectivities and extends Moreno's understanding of co-unconscious processes.

Notes

1 See also Solnit (2009), Nembhard (2014), Steele (2020), and Graeber & Wengrow (2021).
2 The late philosopher Bernard Stiegler describes the sustaining effects of looming catastrophe in the present age as contributing to "collective entropy," suppressing our capacity to symbolize, imagine, and/or creatively think our way into new "religious,

spiritual, artistic, scientific, political movements, manners and styles, new institutions, social organizations, changes in education, in law, in forms of power and of course, changes in the very foundation of knowledge, whether this is in conceptual knowledge or work-knowledge or life knowledge" (Stiegler, 2019, p. 14, cited in Brooks, 2022, p. 24).

3 Anthropologist David Graeber and archaeologist David Wengrow researched the origins of freedom while critiquing the conventional accounts of human social history in their remarkable tome entitled *The Dawn of Everything: A New History of Humanity* (2021). It is impossible to summarize the main points and the anthropological/archeological evidence from which they draw their conclusions here. The authors openly admit that the examples they cite had to be cherry-picked (given the span of time researched) and their interpretations are speculative. Their rigorous scholarship used in support of what they are calling "social freedom" remains compelling. This is especially true in light of what recent Indigenous, African American, and Mexican American histories in the United States are revealing about the mutual aid–based groups and societies discussed later in the chapter.

4 Discussed in length are Eurasia's first urbanites in Mesopotamia, the Indus valley, Ukraine, China, and the American Southern hemisphere (Mesoamerica) where cities were built without a monarchy. Pre-Columbian capitals such as Teotihuacan or Tenochtitlan dwarf the earliest-known cities in China and Mesopotamia. Mega-sites in areas that are known today as Ukraine and Moldova (first discovered in the 1970s) with contemporary names of Taljanky (largest known), Maidentske, and Nebelivka existed prior to 4100 to 3300 BC. The earliest-known sites were in Mesopotamia (fourth and early third millennia BC) and were larger in area. The terrible irony of the current Russian–Ukrainian war is that it is occurring on the very soil that four millennia ago exemplified a civilization that was based on social liberty.

5 From this point forward, we mostly use the term "Quest" instead of "Project Quest."

6 Sarah Schulman relays the experiences of ACT UP activists in New York City in her recent book *Let the Record Show: The Story of How Activists and Scientists Tamed AIDS*. She states: "As a result, all of us were frustrated and fighting for our lives. those with and without power leveraged energy, currency, connection, assertion, insistence, and imagination to transform AIDS" (2021, p. 24).

7 In 1996, a major scientific breakthrough in HIV medicine occurred with the introduction of highly active antiretroviral therapy (HAART) that quickly became a standard of care in the U.S. In the following years, AIDS-related deaths declined dramatically among white patients. Another crisis loomed as the prevalence of AIDS was rising dramatically in minority communities, spawning efforts to increase funding and boost distribution of care. See HRSA Ryan White HIV/AIDS Program A Living History (timeline): https://ryanwhite.hrsa.gov/livinghistory/living-history-timeline#date1996

8 In Chapter 9, Robin closely explores Jungian arts-based research (JABR) design as an innovative approach that is inclusive, open ended, and not owned by the researcher (Rowland & Weishaus, 2021). JABR is an inter- and intra-psychic relational methodology that produces new ways of understanding what it means to be human. We may contrast JABR with scientific inquiry, which dominates mainstream psychology today and has done for over a century since the inception of psychoanalysis.

9 The term "mutual aid" was brought into public use in essays first published at the turn of the 20th century by a Russian anarchist and philosopher, Prince Pyotr Alexeyevich Kropotkin. He was interested in the mutually beneficial cooperation and reciprocity in human societies and within the animal kingdom. His work is considered a crucial catalyst in the scientific study of cooperation as well as a basis for later development of various forms of social activism, demanding transformative change from

the grassroots. See Kropotkin, *Mutual Aid: A Factor in Evolution* (1902/2021). We discuss Kropotkin further in Chapter 1.

10 Dean Spade concisely and concretely defines how mutual aid builds solidarity and promotes grassroots-based collective action within communities during a crisis in his book, *Mutual Aid: Building Solidarity During This Crisis (and the Next)* (2020). Spade's perspective is intended to be a pragmatic manual for activism of all kinds during our present era of sustained catastrophe and accelerated change, without regard to social and eco justice. While his focus is not clinical, he cogently elaborates the key characteristics required to develop a climate where activist movements cohere through solidarity, mutuality, consensus in decision making, and self-determinism. Many of the key elements Spade describes are relevant to how psychotherapy groups may thrive even though the aim of therapy groups is self-development within a group climate and not directed towards a specific activist project (social justice, climate change, systemic racism, etc.).

11 Contemporary critiques consider how traditional psychoanalysis is infantalistic, decontextualizing, apolitical, hierarchical, universalizing, uses the psychology of the individual to explain group phenomenon, siloed, individualistically focused, and hierarchical (Cushman, 1995; Watkins; 2019; Wu, 2013; Gaztambide; 2019; Brooks, 2023; Layton, 2023).

12 These ideas were discussed during an International Association of Jungian Studies Zoom "Town Hall" meeting on September 9, 2023, especially during Peter Dunlap's commentary. See Dunlap (2008) and subsequent works for inspiring insights and experiences of community building.

13 The use of mutuality between patient and analyst within a psychoanalytic context was introduced by feminist psychoanalyst Jessica Benjamin in the 1980s. See Benjamin, *The Bonds of Love: Psychoanalysis, Feminism, and the Problem of Domination* (1988). This was a dramatic shift from the traditional stance of top-down authority and holder of truth that has dominated demagogic psychoanalytic stances into our present era. Graham Harriman discusses Benjamin's contribution to his clinical orientation in Chapter 5. Robin incorporates Jungian thought into her Chapters 6 and 9. Jung's relational stance included a self-to-self and self-to-other engagement of the personal and collective psyche that she extends in her psychodramatic work with groups.

14 The psychology of radical healing for People of Color and Indigenous individuals has been developed in the United States, which reaches beyond individual approaches to cope with racial oppression (French et al., 2020). This framework builds on social justice education and activism as a form of healing transformation that integrates elements of liberation psychology, black psychology, ethnopolitical psychology, and intersectionality theory. Daniel José Gaztambide, in his recent work *From Freud to Liberation Psychology: A People's History of Psychoanalysis* (2019), formulates a psychoanalytically informed theory of race, class, and oppression. His work attempts to integrate the central tenets of the relational school of psychoanalysis, particularly the work of Jessica Benjamin, into a broader liberatory theoretical vision for a psychoanalysis of the people. Gaztambide's study traces psychoanalytic ideas alongside the work of social justice giants such as Frantz Fanon, Paulo Freire, and Ignacio Martín-Baró. Mary Watkins has been a leading voice in liberation psychology for many decades. She is the co-founder of the Community, Liberation, Indigenous, and Eco-Psychologies graduate specialization at the Pacifica Graduate Institution. Her works powerfully critique psychology and psychoanalysis and the oppressive systemic processes at large while offering liberatory alternatives in the ways we might consider embracing (Watkins & Shulman, 2008; Watkins, 2019).

References

Adams, T., Jones, S. H., & Ellis, C. (2015). *Autoethnography: Understanding Qualitative Research*. New York: Oxford University Press.

Anzaldúa, G. (1987). *Borderlands/La Frontera: The New Mestiza*. San Francisco, CA: Aunt Lute Books.

Belkin, M., & White, C. (2020). *Intersectionality and Relational Psychoanalysis: New Perspectives on Race, Gender, and Sexuality*. New York: Routledge.

Benjamin, J. (1988). *The Bonds of Love: Psychoanalysis, Feminism, and the Problem of Domination*. Toronto: Random House.

Brooks, R. M. (2023). *Catastrophe, Psychoanalysis and Social Change*. New York: Routledge.

Christakis, N. (2019). *Blueprint: The Evolutionary Origins of a Good Society*. New York: Little, Brown Spark.

Crenshaw, K. (1989). Demarginalizing the Intersection of Race and Sex: A Black Feminist Critique of Antidiscrimination Doctrine, Feminist Theory and Antiracist Politics. *University of Chicago Legal Forum*, 1(8), 139–167.

Comas-Diaz, L. (2007). Ethnopolitical Psychology: Healing and Transformation. In E. Aldarondo (Ed.), *Advancing Social Justice Through Clinical Practice*, pp. 91–118. Mahwah, NJ: Erlbaum.

Cushman, P. (1995). *Constructing the Self, Constructing America: A Cultural History of Psychotherapy*. Lebanon, IN: Da Capo Press.

Denver Principles (1983). ACT UP Historical Archive. https://actupny.org/documents/Denver.html. Accessed August 10, 2019.

Dunlap, P. (2008). *Awakening Our Faith in the Future: The Advent of Psychological Liberalism*. New York: Routledge.

Dykstra, W. (2014). *Conscientisation and the Ontology of Personhood in Latin American Liberation Psychology*. History & Philosophy of Psychology, 15(1), 1–11.

Freire, P. (1994). *Pedagogy of the Oppressed*. Cambridge, MA: Harvard University Press.

French, B. H., Lewis, J. A., Mosley D. V., Adames, H. Y., Chavez-Dueñas, N. Y., Chen, G. A., & Neville, H. A. (2020). Toward a Psychological Framework of Radical Healing in Communities of Color. *The Counseling Psychologist*, 48(1), 14–46.

France, D. (2016). *How to Survive a Plague: The Story of How Activists and Scientists Tamed AIDS*. New York: Alfred A. Knopf.

Frosh, S. (2003). Psychosocial Studies and Psychology: Is a Critical Approach Emerging? *Human Relations*, 56, 1547–1567.

Frosh, S. (2015). *Psychosocial Imaginaries: Perspectives on Temporality, Subjectivities, and Activism*. (S. Frosh, Ed.). New York: Palgrave Macmillan.

Frosh, S. & Baraitser, L. (2008). Psychoanalysis and Psychosocial Studies. *Psychoanalysis, Culture & Society*, 13, 346–365.

Gaztambide, D. J. (2019). *A People's History of Psychoanalysis: From Freud to Liberation Psychology*. New York: Lexington Books.

Giacomucci, S. (2021). *Social Work, Sociometry, and Psychodrama: Experiential Approaches for Group Therapists, Community Leaders, and Social Workers*. Singapore: Springer.

Gill-Peterson, J. (2018). *Histories of the Transgender Child*. Minneapolis, MN; London: University of Minnesota Press.

Graeber, D. & Wengrow, D. (2021). *The Dawn of Everything: A New History of Humanity.* New York: Farrar, Straus and Giroux.

Halkitis, P. (2015). *The AIDS Generation: Stories of Survival and Resilience.* New York: Cambridge University Press.

Hancock, A. M. (2016). *Intersectionality: An Intellectual History.* New York: Oxford University Press.

Hartman, T. (2021). *The Hidden History of American Healthcare: Why Sickness Bankrupts You and Makes Others Insanely Rich.* Oakland, CA: Berrett-Koehler Publishers, Inc.

Hook, D. (2008). *Six Moments in Lacan.* London; New York: Routledge.

Hooks, bell (2014). *Feminist Theory: From Margin to Center.* New York: Routledge.

HRSA Ryan White HIV/AIDS Program: A Living History (n.d.). https://ryanwhite.hrsa.gov/livinghistory/living-history-timeline#date1996. Accessed November 1, 2022.

Jones, M. S. (2020). *Vanguard: How Black Women Broke Barriers, Won the Vote, and Insisted on Equality for All.* New York: Basic Books.

Kropotkin, P. (1902/2021). *Mutual Aid: A Factor in Evolution.* Manchester, NH: Extending Horizon Books.

Leavy, P. (Ed.). (2018). *Handbook of Arts-Based Research.* New York and London: The Guilford Press.

Lu, K. (2013). Can Individual Psychology Explain Social Phenomena? An Appraisal of the Theory of Cultural Complexes. *Psychoanalysis, Culture & Society*, 18(4), 386–404.

Martín-Baró, I. (1994). *Writings for a Liberation Psychology.* Cambridge, MA: Harvard University Press.

Moreno, J. L. (1953). *Who Shall Survive: Foundations of Sociometry, Group Psychology and Sociodrama.* Beacon, NY: Beacon House Inc.

Nembhard, J. (2014). *Collective Courage: A History of African American Cooperative Economic Thought and Practice.* University Park, PA: The Pennsylvania State University Press.

Ordóñez, E. (2021). *Ancestry: The Deep Field of Reality.* Quechelah Publishing.

Pycior, J. L, (2014). *Democratic Renewal and the Mutual Legacy of US Mexicans.* College Station, TX: A&M University Press.

Saban, M. (2020). Simondon and Jung: Rethinking Individuation. In C. McMillian, R. Main, & D. Henderson (Eds.), *Holism: Possibilities and Problems*, pp. 91–97. London and New York: Routledge.

Schulman, S. (2021). *Let the Record Show: A Political History of Act Up New York, 1987–1993.* New York: Farrar, Straus and Giroux.

Schwartz, W. (1959). Group Work and the Social Scene. In A. J. Kahn (Ed.), *Issues in American Social Work*, pp. 110–139. New York: Columbia University Press.

Stiegler, B. (2019). *The Age of Disruption: Technology and Madness in Computational Capitalism* (Daniel Ross, Trans.). Medford, MA: Polity Press.

Spade, D. (2020). *Mutual Aid: Building Solidarity During a Crisis (and the Next).* New York and London: Verso.

Solnit, R. (2009). *A Paradise Built in Hell: The Extraordinary Communities That Arise in Disaster.* New York: Viking.

Steele, M. (2020). *Indigenous Resilience.* https://papers.ssrn.com/sol3/papers.cfm?abstract_id=3357805. Accessed December1, 2022.

Rowland, S. (2023). Jungian Arts-Based Research (JABR): What It Is, Why Do It, and How. *Journal of Analytical Psychology*, 68(2), 436–439.

Rowland, S. & Weishaus, J. (2021). *Jungian Arts-Based Research and the Nuclear Enchantment of New Mexico.* New York: Routledge.

Ruiz, E. R. (2020). Between Hermeneutic Violence and Alphabets of Survival. In A. J. Pitts, M. Ortega, & J. Medina (Eds.), *Theories of the Flesh: Latinx and Latin American Feminisms, Transformation and Resistance*, pp. 204–219. New York: Oxford University Press.

Watkins, M. (2019). *Mutual Accompaniment and the Creation of the Commons.* New Haven, CT: Yale University Press.

Watkins, M. & Shulman, H. (2008). *Toward Psychologies of Liberation.* New York: Palgrave Macmillan.

Whittingham, M., Lefforge, N., & Marmarosh, C. (2021). Group Psychotherapy as a Specialty: An Inconvenient Truth. *Group Psychology and Group Psychotherapy*, 74(2), 60–66.

Wright, C. (2014). *Workers Cooperatives and Revolution: History and Possibilities in the United States.* Bradenton, FL: BookLocker.com.

Wu, K. (2013). Can Individual Psychology Explain Social Phenomena? An Appraisal of the Theory of Cultural Complexes. *Psychoanalysis, Culture & Society*, 18, 386–404.

Part I

Scientific, Activist, Historical, and Psychological Roots of Mutual Aid

Chapter 1

Scientific Perspectives of Mutual Aid and Survival Activism

Robin McCoy Brooks

Scientific Perspectives: Pyotr (Peter) Kropotkin: Mutuality and Cooperation

The term "mutual aid" was first brought into public use and popularized in the many essays, books, and pamphlets published at the turn of the 20th century by a Russian anarchist, philosopher, and scientist, the revolutionary Prince Pyotr Alexeyevich Kropotkin.[1] His life story through his own words and in the eyes of biographers underscore the degree to which his scientific studies, socio-political notions, and acts of rebellion against the state were bound to his place in history, the social unions he formed (including with animals), and his psycho-social-genetic make-up (Christakis & Fowler, 2011).[2] Kropotkin acted as a bridge between completely different groups of people, ideas, geographic areas, and social classes.[3] His classic interdisciplinary approach to scholarship was typical to the era in which he was born. He would fuse metaphysical and political questions with scientific claims, while his message was specifically anarchist.

One has only to read Kropotkin's introduction to the principal scientific offering *Mutual Aid: A Factor of Evolution* (1902) to grasp his passion for collaboration. He boldly spoke of the relationship of animal love and biological instinct, riding the wave of the zeitgeist or even anticipating the newly emerging fields of psychology and psychoanalysis:

> The book begins with a hymn to Love, and nearly all its illustrations are intended to prove the existence of love and sympathy among animals … It is not love to my neighbor—whom I often do not know at all—which induces me to seize a pail of water and to rush toward his house when I see it on fire … It is a feeling infinitely wider than love, or personal sympathy—an instinct that has been slowly developed among animals and men in the course of an extremely long evolution, and which has taught animals and men alike to … borrow from the practice of mutual aid and support, and the joys they can find in social life.
>
> (Kropotkin, 1902, p. 4)

DOI: 10.4324/9781003386339-3

Kropotkin's interest in mutually beneficial cooperation and reciprocity in human societies was based on the vast field research he conducted as a young man in the remote reaches of Eastern Siberia and Northern Manchuria. Over a five-year odyssey, he traveled over 50,000 miles by foot, boat, cart, horseback, and steamers across unmapped areas, eventually redrawing the map of the Amur region of far northeastern Asia (Harman, 2011). Along the way, he lived and worked with the different peoples he encountered: tribal peoples, prisoners, and villagers.

Having read Darwin's *On the Origin of Species* (originally published in 1859), which emphasized the fierce struggle among species members to survive, Kropotkin was surprised to instead witness the collaboration of wolves coming together to hunt in packs, birds assisting each other in nestbuilding, fallow deer marching in unison at river crossings, and horses forming protective rings in order to guard against predators (Kropotkin, 1902, p. 4). These experiences would later form the basis of arguments *for* an evolutionary emphasis on *mutuality and cooperation* instead of competition and hierarchy (dominance), as asserted by social Darwinists.

In the conclusion of *Mutual Aid*, Kropotkin summarizes his key points regarding progressive evolution:

> In the animal world we have seen that the vast majority of species live in societies, and that they find in association the best arms for the struggle for life: understood, of course, in its wide Darwinian sense – not as a struggle for the sheer means of existence, but as a struggle against all natural conditions unfavorable to the species. The animal species... in which individual struggle has been reduced to its narrowest limits... and the practice of mutual aid has attained the greatest development... are invariably the most numerous, the most prosperous, and the most open to further progress. The mutual protection, which is obtained in this case, the possibility of attaining old age and of accumulating experience, the higher intellectual development, and the further growth of sociable habits, secure the maintenance of the species, its extension, and its further progressive evolution. The unsociable species, on the contrary, are doomed to decay.
>
> (Kropotkin, 1902, p. 145)

Kropotkin's observations of cooperation among species in the wild, in addition to Indigenous peoples and other pre-authoritarian remaining communities in the Russian far east, allowed him to conclude that not all human societies were based on coercive dominance and competition, as were those he noted in industrialized Europe. It is important to add that Kropotkin did not disavow competitive and/or aggressive drives in human beings; rather, he claimed such a view reduced evolution to its "narrowest limits."

Kropotkin was one of the first to refute the idea of "survival of the fittest" put forward by the academics of the 19th century who were heavily under the influence of Neo-Darwinist ideas that sought to justify both capitalism and imperialism. He advocated for a society that was free from hierarchical authoritarian institutions (such as the state and Church), claiming they stifled human creativity and impeded the propensity towards cooperation. Thus, Kropotkin became a radicalized proponent of worker-run enterprises, self-governing communities, and volunteerism, so much so that he was arrested twice and exiled from Russia until after the Russian Revolution in 1917. These basic ideas were central to the formation of mutual aid societies, groups, and fraternities that were simultaneously forming in other parts of the world discussed below.

Critics generally laud the overall scientific basis of Kropotkin's research for not only providing a contribution to the theory of evolution but also in providing a scientific foundation to anarchist theory (Avrich, 1988, p. 59). [4] As such, his political philosophy and actions disavowed the hierarchical forms of governments, institutions, and organizations, including economic policies (capitalism) that maintained coercive dominance over resources by a few over the many (Suisse, 2019). Kropotkin's works are considered a crucial catalyst in the scientific study of cooperation as well as a basis for later development of various forms of social activism that demand transformative change from the grassroots.

The Norm of Group Mutuality

The study of human evolutionary genetics blew up in the second half of the 20th century, encouraging exciting cross-disciplinary discoveries that served to deepen or hone earlier suppositions advanced by Kropotkin and others. Nicholas Christakis' *Blueprint: The Evolutionary Origins of a Good Society* (2019) is a compilation of studies from Yale University's Human Nature lab, which Christakis directs. The contributors' research draws on findings in social science, evolutionary biology, neuroscience, genetics, and network science, in addition to their own studies. Christakis makes the startling conclusion that natural selection has given us the capacity to form "good societies" in spite of humanity's violent propensities to dominate others throughout a large part of history. Christakis attributes these capacities to what he terms a "*social suite*" of features that are at least "partially encoded" in our genes.

These universal, social features have evolutionary origins and influence how groups and social networks function *across cultures* (Christakis, 2019, pp. 12–18). The social suite "universals" include the ability to recognize individual identity, make friends and social networks, relate to offspring, cooperate, show preferences for one's own group, band together, recognize uniqueness, show kindness, love, and reciprocity in our relationships, teach what we know, prefer mild hierarchy, and even to learn socially (Ibid.).

Christakis and colleague James Fowler coauthored an earlier book entitled *Connected: How Your Friends' Friends' Friends' Affect Everything You Feel, Think, and Do* (2011), which establishes the importance of friendships (in the social suite) that nourish other social connections and networks, thus enhancing our propensity for reciprocity and cooperation. Altruism, they hold, is a key predicate for the formation and operation of social networks (Christakis & Fowler, 2011, pp. 296–300). Altruism and reciprocity (aspects of mutual aid) and some degree of emotional positivity (such as love and happiness) are critical for the emergence of social networks and can further *spread through them* (Christakis & Fowler, 2011, p. 296). Altruistic people, in other words, tend to hang out with other altruistic people.

In a later study, Yale Human Nature Lab found that working-class Americans were more likely to rely on friends and neighbors for practical help than were the middle or upper classes. Those who are more affluent tend to rely on formal institutions such as therapists, coaches, colleagues, mentors, and professional advisors, remaining in silos of sameness (Christakis, 2019, p. 247). Those on the fringes of a network have fewer ties and access to fewer resources than those in the center with more ties. The authors correlated positional inequality to patterns of access that are manifestly unjust based on a hierarchical society with socio-political characteristics that stratify and divide the classes (Christakis & Fowler, 2011, p. 300).

Where we are positioned in our social networks may not be our choice, but it also depends on the choices of others around us. If you are wanting to find a new job, healthcare resource (such as where to find a vaccine), therapist, housing, public goods, etc., your chances of being treated with care depends on how well connected you are to those around you, and who, in turn, they are connected to. Friends influence many domains of our lives (physical health, emotions, partner choice, voting patterns, health, access to resources).

At the end of their book (in a section entitled "Reading Group Guide"), Christakis and Fowler summarize their findings for what we can do to spread out our friends and enliven our social networks (edited and paraphrased):

1 Make good behavior visible. We copy each other.
2 Social network equality systems are more altruistic. Social network inequality is an important problem because those on the edges have fewer resources, and those who are well connected have exponentially more access and do not share.
3 Bad things can also spread through social networks but if the overall personal connection is positive each friend makes us healthier and happier... don't dump your friends who do things you don't want to copy; instead, work on influencing them to change.
4 Friends strongly influence us in many domains of our lives – positively and negatively, such as in physical health, emotions, choice of partner, and political opinions.
5 Where you live matters. Your next-door neighbors have a special effect.

(Christakis & Fowler, 2011, pp. 2–4)

Falling into Mutuality

Based on these findings, we can appreciate how crucial it was when Lusijah acted on her insight to form a community *of care* for those who were isolated and living with an HIV-positive diagnosis. They were located on edges of social networks that were neither altruistic nor egalitarian because they were already marginalized: they were most likely gay and now they were infected. Lusijah reached out to her friends, colleagues, and certain family members for help. Her friends (and colleagues), and then their friends' friends, began to build a diversified social network that would ultimately benefit all of us because there were many essential resources. Tangible resources include such things as having a place to live, food, medical care, and transportation. Intangible resources have to do with empathy, respect, reliability, mutuality, and other dynamics that are part of an egalitarian/altruistic social network. The Project Quest (henceforth referred to as Quest) community naturally grew into a mutual aid environment. The impulse to make friends may be written in our DNA. Trauma, shock, and adversity can awaken the agency to do so (Solnit, 2009; Brooks, 2022).

In one study conducted across societies, Christakis found that the most prevalent characteristics of friendships are (by far) mutual aid, positive affect, and equality (the fair distribution of resources and influence) (Christakis, 2019, pp. 244–248).[5] The structure of social networks we form and are formed by begins from our dyadic friendships and our genes. Christakis (2019, p. 198) persuasively argues that while kinship bonds are important, genetic studies suggest that our social networks in fact contain many unrelated individuals who set the stage for cooperation and friendship that is foundational to living in a diversified world versus a segregated one. In other words, for the sake of forming friendships, this sort of diversified mutuality is important and preferable to a uni-cultural tribalism.

Studies show that people choose friends and form groups and networks with a propensity for an in-group bias (one characteristic of the social suite) that can foster ethno-centrism (or other sameness criteria) and discrimination against out-group members (Christakis, 2019, pp. 266–280). The preference for one's own group is also a universal across cultures even though it may be an arbitrary and meaningless bias. Furthermore, individuals studied were often unaware of their in-group biases. Cohesion is spawned by what social workers have coined the "we are all in the same boat" affect because group members share a certain fate (Gitterman & Shulman, 2005). Hidden benefits to in-group favoritism include the enhancement of self-interest, self-esteem, and group identity characteristics that foster the expectation of mutual aid. Our predisposition for in-group preference can also promote a sense of solidarity towards a shared aim beginning with survival. It can also reinforce the divisiveness that promotes exclusion and social injustices. We discuss ways to eradicate such injustices in Chapter 3.

On the other side, being part of a group that has a shared norm of mutuality can foster cooperation *even with strangers*, if, Christakis states, strangers are seen as "one of us" (Christakis, 2019, p. 268).[6] But how can restoration between disparate factions transcend the benefits for in-group bias that are part of our evolved psychology and facilitate cooperation on a larger social network scale? One answer, Christakis identifies, is to share a common enemy, fostering a more *informal* sense of solidarity.

Christakis, however, offers a distinct perspective. "Experiments show," he states, "that positive relations between conflicting groups can only be restored if "super-ordinate" goals of interest to all the groups are in place (Christakis, 2019, p. 269). Yale researchers (in collaboration with Christakis) asked if in-group bias and cooperation could arise without competition between groups.[7] Put another way, they wondered, *how we can have positive feelings about our own group without also having negative feelings about another group?*

They found that developing fluid social dynamics by altering group membership would facilitate the capacity to adopt new successful behavior seen in other groups. Switching groups and being exposed to "strangers," in other words, can contribute to the formation of an egalitarian/altruistic social network that in psychological parlance promotes the individuation of both person and group. Extending these findings to mutual aid groups, we can say that a diverse composition of people (of both in- and out-group) is extremely advantageous.

In any group, there is a constant tension, and this includes those with mutual aid group climates. In times of scarcity, due to competition over resources, ideology, and power, conflict between groups within in-groups can inflame hostility and discrimination towards external groups. We certainly experienced this phenomenon in the many kinds of groups we engaged with in the formation of Quest. In-group bias facilitated an initial sense of cohesion for those who were gay and HIV-positive (the dominant demographic). Others who were not gay, not HIV-positive, and those who were HIV-positive and non-white, were initially on the outside of the dominant demographic. Our open-door policy encouraged fluid social demographics and challenged group dynamics. Struggles over belonging, identity, place, authenticity, privilege, power, the right to live when others died, and basic jealousies were common. These became important features for open, dynamic work in all stages of the group process.

Lusijah and Robin, for example, were often the butt of anti "breeder" jokes initially, as both have children, are white, have privilege, and are not HIV positive. Graham, as a gay man living with HIV symptoms, was a group therapist (status) with privilege (class, race). However, because he was also an active member in the gay and HIV-positive gay community, his presence lent accountability to Lusijah and Robin as allies. In later chapters, we discuss how cohesion was built, alliances were established, trust was formed, transference and counter-transference were worked with, and conflict was handled within mental health mutual aid groups with diverse memberships. As with Christakis above, the common purpose, or *super-ordinate goal*, that brought us together in the first decade of AIDS was the human need to build an empowering social space that resisted the dehumanizing biases about AIDS and gay people perpetuated by society at large.

More recently, we find a similar dynamic that arose acutely following George Floyd's murder in May 2020. This terrible event, among many like it, invigorated one of the largest protest mobilizations against police violence against Black people in U.S. history, including the civil rights marches in the 1960s. White-majority turnout for these protests organized by Black activists in the movement Black Lives Matter *far surpassed* other forms of resistance so far.[8] Otherwise stated, the mass participation of white people moving into (switching groups) Black, brown, and Indigenous political spaces of resistance against police brutality became a "supra-ordinate goal of interest" across racial and class lines.[9]

We have evolved, Christakis claims, to live in differentiated social networks with individuals whom we come to know, care about, learn from, teach, and thereby expand our notions of cooperation. This is how, he concludes, we can live together in the face of all our defects and differences (Christakis, 2019, p. 418). How some groups coalesce into societies that uphold these innate sensibilities is a central topic we develop throughout our book.

Survival Activism and Mutual Aid

We think of mutual aid in the context of survival work, especially when there is collective human suffering and uneven access to resources.[10] This occurs during both short-term crises (such as natural disasters and health crises) and long-term crises (such as systemic marginalization, poverty, and the effects of neo-liberal capitalism). Most recently, mutual aid has gained recognition as it grew to be practiced widely during the COVID-19 pandemic as a way for communities to immediately share resources when governmental and other structures failed (Solnit, 2020). Until recently, use of the term "mutual aid" was primarily limited to social activists, academics, social workers, and psychodrama therapists (Beito, 2000; Solnit, 2009; Nembhard, 2014; Spade, 2020; Giacomucci, 2021). In Chapter 3, we discuss how mutual aid–based community and group work has silently proliferated on the margins of psychology.

From the Trenches: Basic Principles of Mutual Aid

Mutual aid is collective coordination to meet each other's needs. Usually from an awareness that the systems we have in place are not going to meet them.

(Spade, 2020, p. 7)

Mutual aid practices can be *embraced in any group*. It can start in our homes. It can affect how our children are cared for, how we care for animals and our planet, and how health care (including mental healthcare) is practiced. It can affect the ways we work, educate, and relate with our friends and in social networks. And mutual aid determines our engagement in justice advocacy, to name the obvious.

Care is mobilized through the deeply ordinary labor of mutual relating from the perspective that human life is beautiful even in its most unglamorous of times (Spade, 2020). I remember Brice Winters vomiting into a plastic garbage can during an AIDS psychodrama retreat. His body was violently reacting to the medications he was taking. This was not the first or last time a group member needed special attention because of the eruption of sudden bodily symptoms such as fatigue, falling asleep, diarrhea, and explosive farting due to the progression of disease. In Brice's situation, group members spontaneously and tenderly attended to him and his vomit as the session continued. Someone brought him a glass of water and a place was made for him to lie comfortably on the couch with a pillow so that he could participate.

In other words, in mutual aid practice each of us is accepted as we are.[11] Such "micro" expressions contribute to a sense of *cohesion in a group while promoting mutuality and collaboration.* An alliance forms among individuals who need each other with varying degrees of necessity in order to work on significant, common challenges. Reliable reciprocity is the basis of solidarity. *Solidarity is the foundation from which a collective may mobilize in subversive resistance* against the social systems that fail to meet these needs.

Solidarity, not Charity

In contrast to the principles of solidarity, *charity programs* run by many nonprofits, corporations, religious organizations, and governmental agencies are often organized by individuals who do not themselves have experiences as recipients. Contemporary charity is strictly regulated and devised from hard-baked hierarchical systems that determine who receives resources and who is disqualified. Thus, recipients are "othered" shamed, stigmatized, and degraded, and regularly put in double-binds. Think, for example, of the national healthcare system and insurance market that are so complex that we need specialized insurance brokers to decipher terms of care. Methods for deciding who makes the cut often promote the injustices the programs are designed to help (Spade, 2020).We discuss this phenomenon in Part II, where we propose a hybrid mental health and mutual aid model to directly engage the complex and painful realities that psychotherapists, psychologists, counselors, social workers, and public mental health administrators face daily in attempting to do their work.

Mutual aid projects help people *develop skills for decision making, encourage participation and collaboration, and welcome shared leadership because there are different skillsets and different kinds of knowledge* (Spade, 2020). Thus, *leadership is* generally *decentralized and strives to maintain a soft horizontal style* versus a top-down hierarchical authoritarian mandate. Organizing human activity towards a *shared aim* (whatever it is) *without coercion* can for many seem impossible or uncomfortable because so many groups are not organized this way. Often it bucks a trend. We live our entire lives within hierarchical systems where authority figures have exclusive decision-making power from the top down. On the other hand, learned dominance can be unlearned in mutual aid–oriented collective spaces (Ibid.).

Maybe you can remember a mentor, family member, teacher, or colleague whose demeanor somehow encouraged your critical thinking and creativity. Maybe you remember a collective space where you as an individual were respected and valued for who you are and your contributions. It is likely that in such a situation, the feeling of a scarcity of resources was diminished because there was a sense of enough to go around. Perhaps you can remember being a beginner (at anything) and being warmly welcomed, valued, and brought into the fold as you learned. *Information and other resources are shared, not horded.*

"Solidarity Not Charity" is a slogan that emerged from the radical group Common Ground Relief formed to support the residents of Hurricane Katrina in New Orleans in the fall of 2005. The founding of the project was cogently described in the group's *Common Ground Relief Volunteer Handbook*:

> Common Ground Collective was founded on September 5, 2005, just days after Hurricane Katrina swept through the Gulf Coast. Malik Rahim, long-term community organizer, member of the Black Panther Party and Green Party Candidate for New Orleans City Council, put out a call for support as white vigilantes patrolled the streets. Two friends from Austin heeded the call, and came to protect Malik's home in Algiers. Sitting around the kitchen Malik, his partner Sharon and Scott Crow from Austin, looked at the devastation around them, and put out a call for more help. With $50 among them, Common Ground was born.
>
> (Rahim, 2006, p. 4)[12]

Rahim and friends used their social network connections to build a mutual aid collective around a "super-ordinate" *survival goal that transcended racial/class oppression. Volunteers were unpaid and comprised of many races and socio-economic affiliations.* Common Ground would develop a large number of free services and programs for residents of the "predominantly African-America, Native American, Asian and Cajun low-income communities" that were needed in the gap of societal care.[13] These services and projects included roaming medical clinics, building neighborhood computer chains, a tool-lending library, emergency home repair, the distribution of food and supplies, legal support and eviction defense, a women's center, a kids community project, tree services, and garden help. In communities such as this that look out for each other, *nobody is turned away and direct care services are provided as they are needed*, when possible.

Mutual Aid Ethos: Working with Respect

The *Common Ground Relief Volunteer Handbook* is an invaluable artifact that gives us a *pragmatic on-the-ground view into the philosophy and practices* the group devised to orient volunteers to a mutual aid ethos.[14] Noteworthy are the guidelines found in the underlined section of the *Volunteer Handbook* entitled "Working with Respect." Below is a partial reproduction:

1. Our backgrounds have not given many of the tools to build just and sustainable society, so we have to learn from and work with each other to build these visions and practices.
2. Everyone has a piece of the truth, everyone can learn, everyone can teach or share something.
3. Remember all of this (is) a process. What happens along the way is as important as the goals.
4. Respect the work and abilities of others.
5. Take risks within yourself: Participate, give it a chance; have some trust to try on new ideas.
6. Critique inappropriate behaviors NOT the person. Remember, we are ALL still learning.
7. Actively listen to each other: listen to what others are saying before speaking.
8. Be accountable to people and communities we support and yourself.
9. Gives space for MANY voices to be heard.
10. Avoid defensiveness: Be open to legitimate critique of ideas, patterns or behaviors.
11. Mistakes will be made by all of us.
12. Be aware of the effects of your actions on the communities and others around you.
13. Take cues from people in the communities you are working with in the way you interact.

These guidelines sketch out the basic values that are necessary to create a mutual aid climate. They can be amended for your own purposes and used as mutual aid orientation tool in many professional or personal settings. We illustrate how these guidelines may be adapted to clinical and professional mental health settings throughout.

Where People Are, There Will Be Challenges

Having extolled the virtues of mutual aid projects and advocacy movements, we also need to bring to light the underbelly of mutual aid group processes that inevitably arise. Groups often spilt into factions, members come and go, tensions rise, and short-term projects can have a life span that fizzles out or fails precipitously for an infinity of reasons.[15] Furthermore, there is no such thing as a pure mutual aid practice. For a variety of reasons, at different times a point person, meaning one in a structure of horizontal leadership, may need to assume a stronger decision-making position. Reasons for this include a need for group process management that arises because of a program structure adjustment, a crisis, policy changes and clarification, the struggle for power, and control, to name a few examples. Sometimes the basic aims of collectives are both egalitarian and hierarchical at the same time, and thus potentially conflicting forms are hard baked into their organizational structures. Examples include various cooperative structures, fraternal societies, mental health groups including community psychology, nonprofits, professional boards, and labor unions (Beito, 2000; Wolff, 2012; Nembhard, 2014; Steinberg, 2014; Pitkin, 2022).

Basic competencies must be developed within the various stages of mutual aid group formation, whether it is activist focused or has other purposes. These competencies include: dealing with the power struggles coming from inside and outside the community; dealing with internal dissension through collaboration; managing and modeling constructive and necessary disagreement; dealing with leader or project failure; developing effective decision-making processes; developing ways of distributing influence; cultivating a culture of group participation; managing conflicts that arise with in-group and out-group biases (race, gender, status etc.); learning how to listen; learning how to express one's needs; learning how to think critically on one's feet; learning how to collaborate; learning how to have generative conflict and make repairs; developing and valuing transparency versus a super-hero facade (leaving our cape at the door); managing inevitable sexual tensions; regulating workload; emotional regulation; learning how to include and welcome new people; developing team-building skills; learning how to delegate and share responsibility; learning how to engage with difference; developing systems of sharing information; building meeting facilitation skills; managing burnout; incorporating play; dealing with divisive group-splitting maneuvers and destructive gossip; learning how to ask for and receive help; incorporating joy; dealing with big feelings that arise in crisis situations such as grief, depression, disappointment, loss, rejection, failure, death, danger, oppression, trauma, and horror.[16]

It takes time to establish the groundwork for a mutual aid culture when you consider how people today are socially trained and habituated to function under hierarchical systems driven by top-down management. Consider also how our predisposition for in-group preference is challenged in inclusive systems. Furthermore, the psycho/social weight of trans-generational trauma sustained by the dehumanizing systems of social injustice affects a whole community. Ongoing socio/political assaults can deflate a sense of purpose, hope for change, or the *spirit of resilience*.[17] How we understand the inter-relationship between mutual aid and resiliency is the topic of the next section.

Resilience and Mutual Aid

Contemporary resilience theory draws on and informs other disciplines such as disaster response, activism, collective and individual trauma, political theory, ecology, business, anthropology, biology, and sociology (Steele, 2020). The research varies on how to define what resilience is and how it can be applied to persons and systems.

Kirmayer, Sehdev, Whitley, Dandeneau, and Isaac conclude that resiliency occurs at multiple levels such as that of the individual, family, community, nation, or global system, including the ecosystem (Kirmayer et al., 2009, p. 63). The Stockholm Resilience Centre (2015) conducted an interdisciplinary, concise study of resilient social-ecological systems, arriving at a similar conclusion. The Centre defines resilience as:

> … the capacity of a system, be it an individual, a forest, a city or an economy to deal with change and continue to develop. It is about how humans and nature can use shocks and disturbances like a financial crisis or climate change to spur renewal and innovative thinking.
>
> (Stockholm Resilience Centre, 2015)

This definition maintains a multi-dimensional view of resilience that includes the individual and their other environments as they interdependently deal with systemic "shocks" in such a way that opens up an opportunity to meet the moment innovatively. *Social resilience* is further defined as "the ability of human communities to withstand *and recover* from stresses such as environmental change or social, economic or political upheaval" (Stockholm Resilience Centre, n.d.; my emphasis). There are elements of both recovery and innovation in this definition.

Zolli and Healy make a distinction between *resilience and recovery*. Recovery is characterized as an ability to return to an original state after taking in the unforeseen disruptions (Zolli & Healy, 2012, p. 13). They critique and clarify this point by stating:

> In their purest expression, resilient systems may have no baseline to return to – they may reconfigure themselves continuously and fluidly to adapt to ever-changing circumstances while continuing to fulfill their purpose.
>
> (Ibid.)

Returning to an "original state" after a crisis may not be possible, for example if your village has been destroyed, your family has been killed, or you receive a medical diagnosis that forever changes your physicality. Receiving an AIDS diagnosis in the 1980s was a death sentence. Resilience in this case was living with and adapting to the ever-changing circumstances of disease while reconfiguring identity, purpose, and how to live fully while moving towards imminent death (Walker & Salt, 2012, p. xi). More boldly stated, *the ability to creatively retain a deepening sense of identity and purpose amidst catastrophe endures* (Steele, 2020).

Disaster researchers Rao and Greve (2018) introduced the importance of diverse social connectivity to the conversation. Resilient communities, they claim, are better equipped to adapt to disasters if they have organizational diversity already in place with experienced leaders and workers who have dense social connections that allow a community to meet each other in a variety of venues. To be resilient is to be "vitally prepared for adversity which requires improvement in overall capability … generalized capacity to investigate, to learn, and to act, without knowing in advance what one will be called to act upon" (Rao & Greve, 2018, pp. 9–10). Recall Christakis' claim that we have evolved to live in differentiated social networks with individuals whom we come to know, care about, learn from, teach, and thereby expand our notions of cooperation. These social sensibilities (innate) are called upon when we pull together with all of our defects, abilities, and differences to collectively act as a form of civic responsibility.

Building on these studies and our experiences, we define *resiliency* as:

1. a capacity for the individual, collective or system to absorb a disruption,
2. and fluidly adapt,
3. by mobilizing renewal and innovative thinking,
4. while preserving and reconfiguring core identity and purpose,
5. without being irretrievably compromised or altered by it.

Seen from this perspective, we argue that the capacity for resilience is enhanced by the practices of mutual aid. Change is made not by individuals but by individuals within a collective, a collective that embraces a kind of radical democracy that is rooted in creative thought and action so that people can participate from a place that makes sense to them (Schulman, 2021). *Mutual aid, as we are describing it throughout this book, becomes a creatively fluid and adaptive strategy for individuals, communities and social systems to build and/ or remain resilient in adverse conditions whose effects may extend beyond our lifetime.*

The many efforts that a grassroots social movement makes towards advancing their quality of life, and ultimately that of a society, may contribute to a larger historic outcome beyond one's own death. Hundreds of thousands of people, for example, died during the onset of the AIDS pandemic while participating in grassroots volunteer movements and/or social services they could not obtain elsewhere (such as Project Quest).

At the same time, collaborative political reactions were gaining traction across the country that would advance public policy, virology, and the human rights movement into the present day (France, 2016; Schulman, 2021). These human rights advancements were also hastened by the emancipatory struggles of people from the Indigenous, African American, and Latinx diasporas in the Global North and South for centuries. This is a topic of the following chapter.

Notes

1 Kropotkin stated that a renowned zoologist, Professor Kessler, gave a lecture entitled "On the Law of Mutual Aid," highlighting his own observations that a progressive evolution of the species is "far more important than the law of mutual contest" (Kropotkin, 1902, p. I3). Kropotkin used this term to later organize his own theories supporting mutuality and cooperation among the species as being central to progressive evolution.

2 See Kropotkin (1899); Miller (1970).

3 Nicholas Christakis and James Fowler wrote a book on the relatively new (or recognized) science of social networks entitled *Connected: How Your Friends' Friends' Friends' Affect Everything You Feel, Think, and Do* (2011). This work informs Christakis's later 2019 work. Christakis and Fowler state: "People are constrained by geography, socioeconomic status, technology, and even genes to have certain kinds of social relationships and to have a certain number of them … and how they affect emotions, sex, health, politics, money, evolution and technology" (Christakis & Fowler, 2011, pp. xv, xvii). At the turn of the 20th century, Jacob Levy Moreno also conducted scientific investigations of social networks he termed sociometry with groups in Europe and later America. Moreno is underrecognized for his sociometric investigations. Applied sociometry is discussed in Robin's Chapters 6 and 9.

4 Critics of Kropotkin's science question his scientific objectivity, which they contend was swayed by subjective preconceptions (Baldwin, 1970; Miller, 1970). Alternatively, see especially "Kropotkin Was No Crackpot" (Gould, 1988). Who cannot smile at this title?

5 Evolutionary psychologists have argued that contagious disease, for example, evokes xenophobia, creating out-group antagonism and weakening bonds of social integration within a group or community (Schaller & Neuberg, 2012; Rao & Greve, 2018, p. 8). We saw evidence of heightened gay xenophobia at the onset of AIDS that contributed to further isolation for those who were gay or diagnosed at the onset of the pandemic.

6 The Black Panther Party, for example, while comprised of predominantly Black (male and female) members, also had ally support (racial, class diversity) as the party grew. As frequently reiterated, the Black Panther Party was not fighting against white people: their fight was against oppression of any kind, perpetuated by white society, especially police brutality (Bloom & Martin, 2016).

7 Christakis collaborated with mathematical biologists Feng Fu and Martin Nowak (Christakis, 2019, pp. 274–282).

8 See the *New York Times* article "Black Lives Matter May Be the Largest Movement in U. S. History" by Buchanan, Bui, and Patel: www.nytimes.com/interactive/2020/07/03/us/george-floyd-protests-crowd-size.html

9 See Louise Erdrich's novel *The Sentence* (2021) for a poignant account of how Native American culture responded to the COVID-19 pandemic, superimposed with the carnage of George Floyd's murder and its aftermath. The protagonist and her people reside in Minneapolis, Wisconsin, the site of Floyd's murder.

10 "Mutual aid is the radical act of caring for each other while working to change the world" (Spade, 2020, p. 8).

11 Moreno poignantly stated it thus: "To each according to what he is … indicating an all-inclusive acceptance of the individual as they are" (Moreno, 1953, p. xxi).

12 The authors of the *Common Ground Relief Volunteer Handbook* are anonymous, yet on page 5 Malik Rahim is identified as the person who is the main visionary behind the project (living in the affected region), becoming an important point person on the ground. I therefore reference the handbook under Rahim's name. https://web.archive.org/web/20071020184228/http://www.commongroundrelief.org/images/Volunteer_handbook_1-9-06.pdf

13 We interchange the terms Black and African American throughout. Not all Black Americans are descendants of enslaved Indigenous African peoples. Indigenous philosophies and cultural practices, while diverse, originate from ancestral lands and are connected to cultural heritage, tribe, and community (Linklater, 2014, p. 25). We interchange Indigenous, Native, Native American, and First Nation peoples throughout, for those for whom the North American continent is their original home. Indigenous people also migrated to what is now known as Southwest United States, Central America, and South America, including the Caribbean (Puerto Rico, Cuba, and the Dominican Republic). We use the term Chicano, Hispanic, Latinx, and Mexican-American interchangeably regardless of geographic location. Latinx is a gender-fluid term and way of referring to people of Latin American descent (and the Caribbean) residing in the U.S.

14 Lawyer and social activist Dean Spade has identified three key elements of mutual aid that can also be applied to our understanding of what is involved in organizing people in activism work. 1) Mutual aid projects meet survival needs and build shared understanding about why people do not have what they need. 2) Mutual aid projects mobilize people, expand solidarity, and build movements that are participatory. 3) Mutual aid projects solve problems through collective action rather than waiting for saviors (the government or others in authority) (Spade, 2020, pp. 9–20).

15 Robin left Project Quest, for example after ten years of volunteering because she was concerned that a newly hired business manager was (in her opinion) mismanaging the money and had assumed an authoritarian position around decision making. Upon reflection, decades later, she can now see that intermingled with typical power struggles, Quest was transitioning from a volunteer-centered mutual aid organization into a traditional nonprofit clinic. The traditional nonprofit system operates from a monetized medical model. Quest was able to maintain aspects of mutual aid–run groups but only in part of the program, and, even so, these groups were compromised. Lusijah describes the benefits of nonprofit provision for marginalized populations, as well as what is lost, in Chapter 7.

16 We have identified many of these challenges from our own group practices, including during the AIDS crisis. We are incredibly grateful for the intellectual contributions of activist Dean Spade, who discusses at length some of the "pitfalls" that inevitably arise in a mutual aid activist culture in *Mutual Aid: Building Solidarity During This Crisis* (2020). Also, see Sara Schulman's book *Conflict is Not Abuse: Overstating Harm, Community Responsibility, and the Duty of Repair* (2016); like Spade, she supports the virtues of conflict and how we can be in productive communication with each other through disagreement.

17 See Paulo Freire, *Pedagogy of the Oppressed*, 1970/2018. We discuss throughout how the effects of individual, collective, and trans-generational trauma manifest in a group process, as well as techniques for building democratic mutual aid systems.

References

Avrich, P. (1988). *Anarchist Portraits*. Princeton, NJ: Princeton Press.

Baldwin, R. N. (1970). *Kropotkin's Revolutionary Pamphlets*. New York: Dover.

Beito, D. (2000). *From Mutual Aid to the Welfare State: Fraternal Societies and Social Services, 1890–1967*. Chapel Hill, NC: The University of North Carolina Press.

Bloom, J. & Martin, W. (2016). *Black Against Empire: The History and Politics of the Black Panther Party*. Oakland, CA: University of California Press.

Brooks, R. M. (2022). *Psychoanalysis, Catastrophe & Social Change*. New York and London: Routledge.

Buchanan, L., Bui, Q., & Patel, J. L. (2020, July 3). Black Lives Matter May Be the Largest Movement in U.S. History. *The New York Times*. www.nytimes.com/interactive/2020/07/03/us/george-floyd-protests-crowd-size.html. Accessed December 12, 2021.

Christakis, N. (2019). *Blueprint: The Evolutionary Origins of a Good Society*. New York: Little, Brown Spark.

Christakis, N. & Fowler, J. (2011). *Connected: How Your Friends' Friends' Friends Affect Everything You Feel, Think, and Do*. New York: Little, Brown Spark.

Darwin, C. (1859). *On the Origin of Species*. London: John Murray.

Erdrich, L. (2021). *The Sentence*. New York: Harper.

France, D. (2016). *How to Survive a Plague: The Story of How Activists and Scientists Tamed AIDS*. New York: Alfred A. Knopf.

Freire, P. (1970/2018). *Pedagogy of the Oppressed*. New York: Bloomsbury Academic.

Giacomucci, S. (2021). *Social Work, Sociometry, and Psychodrama*. Singapore: Springer.

Gitterman, A. & Shulman, L., (2005). *Mutual Aid Groups, Vulnerable & Resilient Populations, and the Life Cycle*. New York: Columbia University Press.

Gould, S. (1988). Kropotkin Was No Crackpot. *Natural History*, 97(7), 12–21.

Harman, O. (2011). *The Price Altruism: George Prince and the Search for the Origins of Kindness*. Boston, MA and New York, W.W. Norton & Company.

Kirmayer, L. J., Sehdev, M., Whitley, R., Dandeneau, S., & Isaac, C. (2009). Community Resilience: Models, Metaphors and Measures. *Journal of Aboriginal Health*, 5(1), 62–117.

Kropotkin, P. (1899). Memoirs of a Revolutionist. *The Anarchist Library*. https://theanarchistlibrary.org/library/petr-kropotkin-memoirs-of-a-revolutionist. Accessed January 20, 2023.

Kropotkin, P. (1902). *Mutual Aid: A Factor of Evolution*. 2021 reprint. Las Vegas, NV: Amazon.

Linklater, R. (2014). *Decolonizing Trauma Work: Indigenous Stories and Strategies*. Halifax: Fernwood Publishing.

Miller, M. (1970). *Kropotkin: Selected Writings on Anarchism and Revolution*. Cambridge, MA: MIT Press.

Moreno, J. L. (1953). *Who Shall Survive? Foundations of Sociometry, Group Psychology and Sociodrama*. Beacon, NY: Beacon House Inc.

Nembhard, J. (2014). *Collective Courage: A History of African American Cooperative Economic Thought and Practice*. University Park, PA: The Pennsylvania State University Press.

Pitkin, D. (2022). *On the Line: A Story of Class, Solidarity, and Two Women's Epic Fight to Build a Union.* Chapel Hill, NC: Algonquin Books.

Rahim, M. (2006). *Common Ground Relief Volunteer Handbook.* https://web.archive.org/web/20071020184228/http://www.commongroundrelief.org/images/Volunteer_handbook_1-9-06.pdf. Accessed November 1, 2022.

Rao, H. & Greve, H. R. (2018). Disasters and Community Resilience: Spanish Flu and the Formation of Retail Cooperatives in Norway. *Academy of Management Journal,* 61(1), 5–25.

Schaller, M. & Neuberg, S. L. (2012). Danger, Disease, and the Nature of Prejudice. *Advances in Experimental Social Psychology,* 46, 1–54.

Schulman, S. (2016). *Conflict Is Not Abuse: Overstating Harm, Community Responsibility, and the Duty of Repair.* Vancouver: Arsenal Pulp Press.

Schulman, S. (2021). *Let the Record Show: A Political History of ACT UP New York, 1987–1993.* New York: Farrar, Straus and Giroux.

Solnit, R. (2009). *A Paradise Built in Hell: The Extraordinary Communities That Arise in Disaster.* New York: Viking.

Solnit, R. (2020, May 14). The Way We Get Through This Is Together: The Rise of Mutual Aid under Coronavirus. *The Guardian.* www.theguardian.com/world/2020/may/14/mutual-aid-coronavirus-pandemic-rebecca-solnit. Accessed June 22, 2022.

Spade, D. (2020). *Mutual Aid: Building Solidarity During This Crisis (and the Next).* Brooklyn, NY: Verso.

Steele, M. (2020). *Indigenous Resilience.* https://papers.ssrn.com/sol3/papers.cfm?abstract_id=3357805. Accessed December 1, 2022.

Steinberg, D. M. (2014). *A Mutual-Aid Model for Social Work with Groups.* New York: Routledge.

Stockholm Resilience Centre (n.d.). Resilience Dictionary. www.stockholmresilience.org/research/resilience-dictionary.html. Accessed September 10, 2023.

Stockholm Resilience Centre (2015). What Is Resilience? www.stockholmresilience.org/research/research-news/2015-02-19-what-is-resilience.html. Accessed November 12, 2023.

Suisse, J. (2019). Education and Non-domination: Reflections from the Radical Tradition. *Studies in Philosophy and Education,* 38(4), 359–375.

Walker, B. & Salt, D. (2012). *Resilience Practice: Building Capacity to Absorb Disturbance and Maintain Function.* Washington, D.C.: Island Press.

Wolff, R. (2012). *Democracy at Work: A Cure for Capitalism.* Chicago, IL: Haymarket Books.

Zolli, A. & Healy A. M. (2012). *Resilience: Why Things Bounce Back.*

Chapter 2

A Brief History of U.S. Mutual Aid Movements

Robin McCoy Brooks

We consider in this chapter how mutual aid has been expressed in the recent history of the United States into the present moment. This often hidden, or repudiated, history may lead us to rethink the nature of human capacities to create social liberatory societies, as well as our indebtedness to the cultures and forgotten knowledge systems of Indigenous, enslaved, occupied, and emigrant societies.[1] The larger questions about what kind of societies are possible in the absence of coercive authority form an over-arching theme.

Alongside its reputation for rugged individualism, unchecked capitalism, and colonializing oppression, the United States has a very rich history of cooperation and communalism. Chris Wright identifies central themes in the history of cooperative uprisings, noting the profound tension between democratic, anti-authoritarian impulses of those who were drawn to mutual aid principles and practices (recalling Kropotkin, Christakis, and Graeber & Wengrow) and the contrary tendency of economic power structures to concentrate on ever-larger and more centralized coercive practices that penetrate the most intimate parts of our lives today (Wright, 2014, p. 71). Mutual aid enterprises and resistance movements against oppression arose from the very heart of this tension amidst a wide swath of peoples.

The intercultural connections between Latinx, African American, Indigenous, European, and Asian cultures go back for centuries and remain a pervasive aspect of life in the American Hemisphere (Ortiz, 2018). Intellectual histories written from the perspectives of Indigenous, Black Americans, Latinx, and other oppressed peoples are slowly coming into the American intellectual mainstream amidst fierce resistance in conservative parts of the country.[2] These perspectives radically liberate us from the familiar stories about U.S. history that have imposed limitations on our understandings of our responsibility to it and how we can imagine a future we can fall in love with.

Contemporary scholars are adapting an *inclusive movement approach* to re-envision an American history that draws on the many overlapping revolutionary traditions that actively challenge pervasive ideologies founded on Euro-white American exceptionalism and racial capitalism. We draw on these

DOI: 10.4324/9781003386339-4

inclusive-movement historical approaches to untangle how methods of resistance are linked to mutual aid practices and are already informing mental healthcare today. In this chapter, we trace the powerful historic currents of mutual aid practices and movements in the U.S. across cultures that arose prior to and after the rise of benevolent associations and fraternal societies at the turn of the 20th century.

Mutual Aid Prior to 1900: An Inclusive Movement Approach

For thousands of years prior to and after European colonization on the North American continent in 1492, Indigenous peoples and nations were already practicing variations of what we are calling mutual aid today. Contemporary scholarship challenges the story of the European conquest of Native Americans. The narrative of this history, seen through the lens of a white colonizer, has dominated U.S. history.[3] Historian Pekka Hämäläinen, for example describes four hundred years of diasporic resistance by the many Indigenous tribes whose strategic, spiritual, and diplomatic maneuvering, either in collaboration with other tribal nations or singularly, fought against white encroachment at every turn to the present day (Hämäläinen, 2022). American empires, he argues, invested political power through the state and bureaucracy in stark contrast to Indigenous nations who invested power in tribal sovereignty and kinship. Hämäläinen describes kinship as:

> … an all-pervasive sense of relatedness and mutual obligations – became the central organizing principle for human life. Kinship was the crucial adhesive that kept people and nations linked together … they opted for more horizontal, participatory, and egalitarian ways of being in the world – a communal ethos available to everyone who was capable of proper thoughts and deeds and willing to share their possessions.
>
> (Hämäläinen, 2022, p. 24)

There is a remarkable democratic and egalitarian statement found in this description. The views and opinions of others are given merit, and mutual care is held as what we would call today a "gold standard." Expertise is derived as a communal experience, subject to changing with life or group (social) circumstances.

Legal historian Michalyn Steele similarly, argues that tribes have largely preserved themselves as distinct peoples, and legal entities, to this day even though American law and policy often violently tramples tribal identity, governance, and culture (Steele, 2020, pp. 313–322). The brute force of the federal government did not compel the majority of Native peoples to abandon their distinct tribalism or beliefs, although it did cause systemic poverty and intergenerational trauma that many tribes are continuing to heal today (Steele, 2020).

Both Hämäläinen and Steele attribute Indigenous resilience to a capacity to retain tribal sovereignty amidst a history of violent oppression. The ability to continue under such harsh conditions is nurtured by long-held traditional and spiritual belief systems, held together by a general communal ethos practiced through the customs and rituals of each tribe. This communal ethos cannot be reduced to what we are calling mutual aid; rather, it informs it.

Martin Luther King, Jr. persuasively argued that the *struggle for civil rights has for over four centuries become a model of democracy for the nation as a whole within the very specter of its impossibility* (King, Jr., 1991). Let us catch our breath from the magnitude of this statement. The history of African American mutual aid practices *began* with the enslavement of African peoples who were separated from their many tribes, clans, and nations by white Americans in 1619. Enslaved Black people continued cooperative practices for over two centuries through the antebellum period (late 18th century to 1865) and after the American Civil War (1961–1965) (Du Bois, 1907). Historian Jessica Gordon Nembhard notes that religious gatherings among slaves were also mutual aid gatherings and channels for collective resistance as they became a base for planning survival strategies (Du Bois, 1898; Curl, 1980; Nembhard, 2014, p. 33),[4] organized resistance, and pooling resources to buy each other's freedom and escape (Du Bois, 1898).

William Still intricately chronicled the design and implementation of escape routes throughout the U.S. and Canada through the underground railroad system. These are examples of highly sophisticated social and economic cooperation among African Blacks and allies (Still, 2019).[5] The underground railroad linked already independent Black communities with one another (Nembhard, 2014, p. 33; Ortiz 2018, pp. 27, 40, 59). Slave fugitives organized communal settlements comprised occasionally of both Black and/or First Nation peoples, wherever slavery existed (Curl, 1980). The first fugitive slave mutual aid communities were recorded in 1830, and they spread throughout the American Midwest and southern Ontario.

The earliest Black community institutions were, in fact, mutual aid societies (Hine et al., 2010). By the end of the Civil War (1861–1865), freed African Americans formed intentional (versus hidden) Black communities that were precursors to formal economic cooperatives. Early cooperatives proliferated and took the form of mutual aid and beneficial societies, fraternal organizations, and collective farms. The first official Black mutual aid society was organized in Newport, Rhode Island in 1780, followed by rapid formation of other societies in the early 1800s in the North and urban areas (Nembhard, 2014). While the first societies were male dominated, Nembhard reports that by 1790, women had established their own societies, sometimes becoming more influential than male-oriented societies well into the 1900s (2014, pp. 43, 50–52, 148–71).[6]

Many people of Mexican origin living in what is now the Southwest United States could not be considered in any sense immigrants because their settlement predates colonization, on the Eastern Shore, by over 3,000 years. Following the Spanish invasion of Central America in the 16th century, a new hybrid race comprised of Indigenous and Spanish blood emerged. Many migrated to, and settled in, parts of their ancestral lands in what is today the U.S. Southwest as early as the 16th century (Anzaldúa, 1987). "For Indians," (Mexican) Gloria Anzaldúa claims, "this was a return to their place of origin" (Ibid. p. 27).

Mexico's resistance to the "illegal" migration of U.S citizens into its northern regions and President James Polk's expansionist agenda resulted in the fateful Mexican–American War (1846–1848). This was initiated by the U.S. invasion of Mexican territories.[7] After Mexico lost the war, the Treaty of Guadalupe Hidalgo was negotiated in 1848, requiring Mexico to relinquish an astonishing *one-third* of its land mass, what are now Texas, New Mexico, Arizona, California, Wyoming, Utah, and Colorado. While Mexicanos who remained in these territories were given "citizenship," legal measures were soon passed to deny most Mexican Americans and their descendants full rights as citizens. Indeed, Mexican (now Mexican Americans) were driven off farms and gold-mining claims, lynched, and ruthlessly assaulted by vigilantes, for many decades.

It is important to note that at the same time, antislavery insurgencies in Haiti, Mexico, and Latin America were also heating up, in what can be seen as an invigorated "hemispheric liberation movement" among Mexicans, African Americans, Native Americans, and abolitionist allies, who were not tied by nationality or contained by sudden artificial borders (Ortiz, 2018). These borderless coalitions inspired anti-imperialist rebellions in Spanish Florida, perpetuated by coalitions of African and Indigenous peoples (Ibid., pp. 36–38). The battle against slavery, in other words, had been percolating across the Americas in movements that rejected three centuries of European colonialization. These movements advocated for the abolition of slavery and the racial caste system in Mexico and elsewhere. Furthermore, alliances between Native Americans, Freed Black Americans, and African slaves were threatening what we refer to today as racial capitalism by providing anti-slavery sanctuaries in the U.S., Canada, and Mexico. This was operationalized through the underground railroad. These sanctuaries were located on land occupied by Indigenous peoples, with limited access to white citizens.[8]

U.S. leaders denigrated these insurgencies by advancing a more rigid framework of "white exceptionalism" that argued that Black people (and other non-white people) did not have the capacity (ability, experience, etc.) to rule. This political propaganda was used to justify the continuing practices of slavery and genocidal removal of American Indians and Mexican occupants from native lands (Ortiz, 2018). Anglo racism against Mexicans, American Indians, free and enslaved Black people, and Chinese immigrants was interwoven into the many laws passed in this period denying basic human rights to each group. These racist laws disallowed basic rights to due process, public assembly, equal access to property and employment, fair wage, and voting rights (Pfaelzer, 2007).

The passage of these laws made it difficult to maintain community-based mutual aid traditions within small towns and barrios for Mexican immigrants and

Mexicans who remained in what had become the U.S. Territory. These traditions had for hundreds of years cultivated cultural solidarity amidst intense pressures to assimilate to a different way of life. Mexican hometown associations and mutual aid societies, or *sociedades mutualistas*, sponsored many cooperative trans-border projects, including product trade, for generations.[9] Prior to the rise of formal labor unions, labor organizations arose that organized work projects performed by its members—a practice that continues to this day (Rivera, 1984, p. 28).

Labor unions were granted the right to exist in the U.S. in 1842, and membership quickly grew in the East among those seeking a working environment that reflected a democratic form of governance (Commons, 1998, p. 565). Following the Civil War, strikes erupted as a response to wage cuts, brought on by an economic depression, resulting in a new surge of union-established cooperativism. While some labor unions were racially integrated (such as the Knights of Labor), most were not. Marginalized groups organized their own unions and labor-supporting organizations (Fink, 2022).

Economic cooperatives emerged as part of a broad-based labor movement. Cooperatives (then and now) are an alternative means of employment because they are companies owned by people who use their services as member-owners.[10] Wright contends that cooperatives were then, and continue to remain, an essential tool to the class struggle in the U.S. and abroad (Wright, 2014, pp. 13–18). Many ethnically and class-diverse peoples have benefited from cooperative ownership and democratic economic participation throughout the history of the United States to the present day. Unions would establish cooperatives in many states prior to the turn of the 20th century, but their popularity dramatically waned due to insufficient financial support and persistent hostility by conventional businesses.[11]

Mutual Aid Movements and Societies into the 20th Century

At the turn of the 20th century, thousands of "fraternal" and other benevolent societies supported essential networks of care, solidifying the labor, cooperative, and social justice movements. These mutual aid approaches proliferated within the absence of a coherent governmental system of welfare provision across racial, cultural, gender, and class differences. Historian David Beito maintains that there is no equivalent today, in American society, for what was then a massive and popular multi-class membership in fraternal orders among wage earners at the turn of the 20th century (Beito, 2000, p 17). Between 1890 and 1920, the U.S. experienced a massive infusion of ethnic and cultural diversity due to the immigration of more than 18 million people, largely from Eastern and Southern Europe. While some societies were racially and/or ethnically integrated, most were not. Black people, Indigenous, Mexican Americans, Caribbean, Jewish, Asian, Russian, Greek, Slovak, Croatian, Irish, Lithuanian, Polish, German, Italian, white, Scandinavian peoples, and women (to name a few) generally formed their own mutual aid societies that reflected distinct cultural values, each having critical distinctions (Beito, 2000, pp. 21–62).[12]

Chinese migration to the United States picked up during the mid-19th century when primarily male manual laborers arrived in the West Coast for work in agriculture, mining, and railroad construction.[13] By 1930, 1.2 million Black Americans migrated to the north. Migrants and immigrants encountered fierce hostility expressed in deeply entrenched racist environments.[14] Trade unions ruthlessly pitted white workers against Chinese, immigrant, Black, and Latinx workers (Liu, 2018). Out of necessity, marginalized groups created formidable social networks for individual and collective protection, and resistance.[15]

By the late 19th century, three types of fraternal societies dominated the scene: secret societies, health and funeral benefit societies, and life insurance societies (Beito, 2000). The common denominator of these organizations was an emphasis on mutual aid and reciprocity. As these societies became more sophisticated, they developed systems of shared values, including the advancement of mutualism, self-reliance, business training, thrift, leadership skills, self-government, and the building of good moral behavior (Beito, 2000, p. 27; Nembhard, 2014, pp. 41, 53). Formal distinctions based on income and class were generally prohibited as membership usually included all economic classes, including the poorest strata of society.

The aims of mutual aid organizations often involved dual political and social welfare agendas. An example can be found in the women's suffragette movement. Mainstream historical accounts often fail to adequately reflect the complex interchanges between white and African American suffragettes at the turn of the 20th century. Black women belonged to a long tradition of women's activism through their involvement with African American–led organizations, antislavery societies, churches, and women's clubs dating back to the early 19th century. By 1905, the National Association of Colored Women (NACW) was established, which included a woman suffrage department by 1908. Nevertheless, Black women were marginalized and excluded as racism permeated white-dominated organizations such as the National American Woman Suffrage Association (NAWSA) (Jones, 2020, pp. 157–160).[16]

Historian Martha S. Jones highlights that Black women's politics were distinct from those of white women. The historical impact of female slavery and the racial devaluation of Black womanhood, especially in the South, created different modes of oppression for racialized women (Zinn & Dill, 1996, pp. 321–331). While both white and Black women would join the suffragette movement in a semblance of solidarity, with the shared aim of obtaining the right to vote, *racial inequality was largely ignored*. The white women's suffragette movement was primarily motivated to gain equal status between white women and men at this time (Thompson, 2002).

Nevertheless, Black women activists such as Mary Church Terrell (and others) persisted in campaigning for equal rights with and separately from the NAWSA, as the outcome of the ratification of the 19th Amendment in 1920 would lead to conditions that were radically different for women of color (Jones, 2020, pp. 155–169). While white suffragettes were dismantling their organization, Black women were preparing to move the struggle for equal rights forward because the 19th Amendment did not eliminate the state laws that suppressed African Americans from voting. These state laws included poll taxes, literacy tests, sexual abuse, and lynching, a reality that continues to this day.

Later in the century, feminists of color such as bell hooks, Kimberlé Crenshaw, and Gloria Anzaldúa (and others) would challenge the historical exclusion of the non-white experience in earlier waves of the feminist movement. They established that the forms of oppression for women of color, the poor, and disabled women are different from the experiences of white women.[17]

Mutual aid organizations became more widespread for people living with disabilities in the 20th century. For centuries, those living with disabilities have been living in a state of forced dependency on family, doctors, and psychiatric hospitals, where decisions were and continue to be made for them. The League of Physically Handicapped was organized in the 1930s in a joint effort to fight for employment in the wake of the Great Depression. In the 1940s, a group of psychiatric patients formed a movement named "We Are Not Alone," supporting patient transition from hospital to the community.[18]

After the Great Depression, mutual aid societies began to decline in membership for a variety of reasons. Beito describes a number of factors that contributed to their decline, including concern for group and personal stability in adverse economic conditions, accusations of corruption within societies, restrictive federal quotas limiting immigrants from Europe, the assimilation of immigrants into mainstream culture, adverse legislation affecting all kinds of insurance, the rise of company pensions and workers' compensation, and changing cultural opinions about the efficacy of mutual aid, family networks, and neighborhood cooperation as solutions to poverty (Beito, 2000; Pycior, 2014, pp. 62–65).

The widespread prevalence of voluntary reciprocity at the turn of the 20th century gave way to impersonal bureaucracies, oligarchic corruption (including in the healthcare system), and grossly inadequate social welfare provisions because their services were appropriated for profit corporation (Hartman, 2021). Mutual aid practices would become more affiliated with coalition building, with their grassroots tributaries flowing into national and international activist movements. These social activist movements have mobilized networks of solidarity and resistance against egregious social and political subjugation into the present day.

Emancipatory Internationalism, and the Creation of Coalitions

The assassinations of Black empowerment leader Malcolm X, in 1965, and mainstream civil rights leader, Martin Luther King, Jr., in 1968 would ignite the rise of liberatory coalitions. These were, and are today, comprised of individuals and communities with overlapping yet distinct social identities, solidified through a shared resistance to the many modes of oppression. For example, in 1969, the Chicago-based Black Panther Party chairman Fred Hampton would form the first anti-racist and anti-classist "Rainbow Coalition" that would unite *The Young Patriots* (organizing poor whites) and *The Puerto Young Lords* (organizing Latinx) with the Black Panthers. As Hampton famously stated: "We got blacks, brown and whites ... we've got a Rainbow Coalition" (Bloom & Martin, 2016, p. 292). Within the same year, Hampton would be ruthlessly murdered in his bed by law enforcement officials, along with Mark Clark who was also in Hampton's apartment.[19] Fourteen years later, presidential candidate Jessie Jackson formed a second Rainbow Coalition that sought to include Native Americans, Asian Americans, youth, disabled veterans, lesbians and gay people, and Jewish Americans to affiliate with African Americans in a joint civil rights struggle.

Activist coalitions in the 1980s and 1990s such as *ACT UP* and *Queer Nation* (and others) pushed the global AIDS pandemic into the political foreground by demanding government intervention (Halkitis, 2015; France, 2016). These and countless other initiatives monumentally advanced the gay rights movement into a human rights movement, thereby challenging people across the country to rethink diversity. These efforts produced more nuanced understandings of gender, race, class, sexuality, disability, religion, and ethnicity in fierce hemispheric liberation movements that continue today.

Ableism, or the social discrimination against people who are disabled, or are perceived as having disabilities, was and is astonishingly prevalent in all strata of society today. If you are a mental health clinician, did your training include working with individuals living with physical (mental health and illness) and invisible disabilities? Are your clinics or offices accessible? In 1990, a group of differently abled protesters and allies gathered on the steps of the U.S. Capitol building, awaiting the passage of the landmark Americans with Disabilities Act (ADA). The legislation was stalled by the over-powering resistance of public transport companies. In an act of profound inspiration and personal sacrifice, some of the protesters threw their wheelchairs, crutches, and walkers aside and *dragged their bodies up the steps* of the U.S. Capitol building, highlighting the necessity for accessibility.[20] This is a poignant moment where empowering resistance met the faces of disempowering greed.

Closing Thoughts

We take the long historical/evolutionary view that ancient and powerful forces are at work, propelling society through cooperation and mutual aid today, often as subversive enterprises. Chapter 3 builds on the significance of the broader history of mutual aid covered in this chapter. Thus, we are better able to grasp and appreciate the legacy from which mutual aid informed group and community practices that emerged in the mental health field. They arose as forms of resistance against what was missing in society but also as a correction to psychology's uncritically held theories and practices. Re-envisioning psychology through the timeless wisdom of mutual practices is a central theme of this book.

Notes

1 More comprehensive analyses of the history of mutual aid are provided by authors that are cited throughout this chapter. Omissions to these stories are ours, alone. "History, despite its wrenching pain, cannot be unlived, but if faced with courage, need not be lived again" (Maya Angelou, *New York Times*, January 21, 1993).
2 See Rivera (1984), Nembhard (2014), Pycior (2014), Bloom & Martin (2016), Jones (2020), and Steele (2020). Nevertheless, book bans against BIPOC and LBGTQ authors continue to persist in U.S. school systems at alarming rates. See National Coalition Against Censorship: https://ncac.org/news/blog/top-10-banned-books-that-changed-the-face-of-black-history
3 Scholars warn us against historical narratives that overly generalize native Americans as a "human Monolith cut from a single-and primordial-cultural cloth," and the tendency to generalize from the study of a single Native nation to provide a comprehensive portrait of traditions, political structures, material culture, and historical experiences (Steele, 2020; Hämäläinen, 2022, pp. xi–xiii).
4 Nembhard (2014, p. 33) notes that these early religious activities predated independent African American churches.
5 William Still was a historian and social activist during the abolitionist movement at the height of the underground railroad efforts in the mid-1800s. Still first published *The Underground Railroad Records* in 1872, as an autoethnographic account of the gripping inner workings of the "the road tracing one of the most successful campaigns of mutual aid based disobedience, in American History." The volume was compiled of firsthand accounts, letters, and anecdotes from those who had escaped from slavery and those, such as Still, who assisted. Novelist Ta-Nehisi Coates introduces the 2019 edition of Still's work. Coates acknowledges that Still's historic account greatly influenced the narrative bones of his novel, *The Water Dancer*, 2019.
6 Kathleen Berkeley furthers this observation by stating: "Black women were often in the vanguard in founding and sustaining autonomous organizations designed specifically to improve social conditions within their respective communities to solve the problems caused by inadequate health care services, substandard housing, economic deprivation and segregated schools" (Berkeley, 1985, p. 184). Martha S. Jones (2020) supports this observation in her research on the long history behind Black women's fight against voter suppression that preceded the ratification of the 19th Amendment and extends to the present day.
7 Mexico was a newly sovereign state having attained its independence from Spain in 1821. The northern region was not a high priority for the central government (due to complex internal political challenges), becoming vulnerable to expansive raids (livestock and looting) by Native American tribes (Comanche, Apache, Navajo), leading to many deaths of the Mexican inhabitants and seriously impacting the stability of the region's agricultural and commercial life. In the United States, the war and resulting treaty drew fierce criticism within the government for its ruthless pursuit, causalities, and expense. This opposition deepened the already sectional divisions within the government. See Rodriguez (2001) and Ortiz (2018).
8 Racial or "slavery capitalism" is a term coined by Cedric Robinson, appropriated from intellectual discourse referencing South Africa's economy under apartheid.

He argues that what made capitalism racial was that racism already permeated in Western society. This was expanded in the colonial process of expropriation, settlement, and white supremacy throughout Europe and its various colonies (Robinson, 2000, p. 3). It is important to note that until recently, U.S. scholarship has generally maintained a hard division between the analysis of capitalism and slavery. New arguments reveal how this artificial division does not hold (Singh, 2017; Brooks, 2022, p. 139; Clegg, 2020).

9 Julie Leininger Pycior gives a robust account in *Democratic Renewal and the Mutual Aid Legacy of US Mexicans* of trans-border (between Mexico and U.S territories) organizing. Organizing efforts ranged from sending money to relatives in Mexico, organizing labor strikes, building alliance networks with grassroot *mutualista* organizations, lobbying against immigration restriction, and building international coalitions to advance various trade policies (Pycior, 2014, pp. 83–100). Mexican immigrant hometown associations have been engaged in trans-border mutual aid for generations. Money sent to Mexico (back home) by immigrants constitutes Mexico's second-largest revenue source (p. 13).

10 Nembhard defines a cooperative as a company owned by the people who use their services. The member-owners create the company to meet particular needs, such as economic or social, to provide a good-quality service at an affordable price and to create an economic contribution to compensate for market failure (2014, pp. 2–3). Many cooperatives, she furthers, formed to address economic, social (mutuality and participation), and ecological sustainability. With others, Nembhard describes the benefits of worker-owned cooperatives and the differences between cooperative entities (Nembhard, 2014, pp. 4–15). See Wright (2014) and Wolff (2014) who view (as does Nembhard for Black Americans) self-directed cooperatives as a cure for capitalism and a way of having democracy at work.

11 Beginning with the Great Depression, a resurgence of economic and self-help cooperativism would reemerge, including agricultural and consumer co-ops that became even more decentralized than in previous periods across racial lines. With the support of government funding, self-help cooperatives surged, organized around a bartering and exchange of goods and services, including labor services, in farms in exchange for food. Nembhard traces the rise and fall of Black economic cooperatives to the present day, claiming that they were, and continue to be, a "necessary expansion of in-group solidarity and cohesion" (2014, p. 32). Mainstream interest in cooperative movements plummeted, with the exception of agriculture, especially in the Northwest, through the 21st century. This is attributed to the end of the New Deal and World War II, and a conservative post-war America (Wright, 2014).

12 See also Tyesha Maddox's (2018) research about the study of the crucial and under-recognized participation of Caribbean immigrant women. Her work considers Caribbean immigrant benevolent associations and mutual aid societies at the turn of the 20th century in the U.S.

13 Chinese immigrants are the third-largest foreign-born group in the U.S. today. In 1882, the Chinese Exclusion Act severely limited further migration as a political response to racist attitudes and pressures, by labor unions. This was repealed in 1943. See Nembhard (2014), Wright (2014), and Ortiz (2018, pp. 118–119, 138–142). Cooperation, and mutual aid has been essential for Asian immigrants coming to the U.S. for the survival and perseverance of these communities facing hostile environments. Collective help took the form of family organizations and benevolent societies. See Yvonne Yen Liu, May 22, 2018, "For Asian Immigrants, Cooperatives Came from Home Country", *Yes!* www.yesmagazine.org/democracy/2018/05/22/for-asian-immigrants-cooperatives-came-from-the-home-country. Accessed January 15, 2023.

14 Julie Leininger Pycior describes, for example, that labor-organizing-based *mutualistas* did not consider immigration status or citizenship as criteria for membership, and, like all Mexican mutual aid–based associations, provided insurance benefits (2014, p. 78). *Mutualistas* have played a prominent role in civil rights and labor movements to this day. One of the most successful of these organizations, in the first half of the 20th century, was *Alianza Nacional México-Americana*, whose many chapters provided legal assistance and funding for victims of racial or class injustice to Mexican Americans. *Alianza* was founded by several *mutualista* groups, and had varied sponsors with its membership coming from the barrios. Pycior notes that by the 1940s, mutualism was considered obsolete, although *Alianza* was running many civil rights programs related to criminal justice, immigration, citizenship, and desegregation into the 1950s.

15 For example, a federation of Chinese mutual aid associations—Chinese Six Companies—responded to racial oppression at the turn of the 20th century. From 1860 to the early 1900s, a number of epidemics sieged the San Francisco Bay area. Public officials scapegoated Chinese-Americans for the spread of the diseases, blaming living conditions and cultural vices for the outbreaks. Local government refused to finance crucial services and raised the cost of treatment for Chinese patients at municipal hospitals. In response, Chinese Six Companies decided to self-fund their own hospital in 1900, named *Tung Wah* Dispensary, the first Chinese-American hospital in the continental United States. This hospital later evolved into the Bay Area Chinese Hospital, which over a century later, during the COVID-19 pandemic, provided a rigorous, and successful response to the crisis, again in the face of fierce anti-Chinese racism (Wang, 2020).

16 In *Vanguard: How Black Women Broke Barriers, Won the Vote, and Insisted on Equality for All* (2020), Jones offers us a rigorous account of the history of the Black women's activism movement, including the right to vote amidst voter suppression that is present today. Jones highlights the lives of key Black women activists: Maria Stewart, abolitionist and suffrage advocate, Frances Ellen Watkin Harper, Mary Church Terrell, community organizer, Fannie Lou Hamer, and Jessie DePriest, to name a few. Burroughs, for example, in addition to voting rights, foregrounded abolishing sexual abuse, the presence of inter-racial cooperation among women, and women having power in the Church within her lifetime (pp. 203–214).

17 See bell hooks (2014) and Gloria Anzaldúa (1987). Kimberle Crenshaw (1989) would introduce the concept and term "intersectionality" in a pair of essays describing the overlapping systems of power that affect those who are most marginalized in society. This concept has been advanced by queer scholarship, and applied to many other fields such as law, politics, education, healthcare, economics, and psychology.

18 See Disability Social History Project (2022): https://disabilityhistory.org/category/disability-rights/ and Lois Curtis (also on this site) in an article on her: www.npr.org/2022/11/05/1134426128/lois-curtis-who-won-a-landmark-civil-rights-case-for-people-with-disabilities-di. Accessed October 5, 2022.

19 A civil lawsuit was later filed in 1982 on behalf of Hampton and Clark's surviving relatives that was later resolved with a financial settlement (Bloom & Martin, 2016, p. 292).

20 See Disability Social History Project (2024).

References

Angelou, M. (1993, January 21). The Inauguration: On the Pulse of Morning. *New York Times*. www.nytimes.com/1993/01/21/us/the-inauguration-maya-angelou-on-the-pulse-of-morning.html. Accessed December 10, 2022.

Anzaldúa, G. (1987). *Borderlands/La Frontera: The New Mestiza*. San Francisco: Aunt Lute Books.

Beito, D. (2000). *From Mutual Aid to the Welfare State: Fraternal Societies and Social Services, 1890–1967.* Chapel Hill, NC: The University of North Carolina Press.

Berkeley, K. C. (1985). Colored Ladies Also Contributed: Black Woman's Activities from Benevolence to Social Welfare, 1866–1896. In W. J. Fraser Jr., F. Saunders Jr., & J. L. Wakelyn Jr. (Eds.), *The Web of Southern Relations*, pp. 181–201. Athens: University of Athens Press.

Bloom, J. & Martin, W. (2016). *Black Against Empire: The History and Politics of the Black Panther Party.* Oakland, CA: University of California Press.

Brooks, R. M. (2022). *Psychoanalysis, Catastrophe & Social Change*. New York and London: Routledge.

Clegg, J. J. (2020). A Theory of Capitalist Slavery. *Journal of Historical Sociology*, 33(1), 74–98.

Coates, T. (2019). *The Water Dancer*. New York: One World.

Commons, J. R. (1998). *History of Labour in the United States, Vol. I.* New York: Beard Books.

Crenshaw, K. (1989). Demarginalizing the Intersection of Race and Sex: A Black Feminist Critique of Antidiscrimination Doctrine, Feminist Theory and Antiracist Politics. *University of Chicago Legal Forum*, 1(8), 139–167.

Curl, J. (1980). *History of Worker Cooperation in America: Worker Cooperation or Wage Slavery: Co-ops, Unions, Collectivity, and Communalism from Early America to the Present.* Toledo, OH: Homeward Press.

Disability Social History Project (2022). Louis Curtis, Disability Rights Activist Who Won a Landmark Civil Rights Case (1967–2022). https://disabilityhistory.org/category/disability-rights/. Accessed January 2, 2023.

Disability Social History Project (2024). Moments in Disability History. https://disabilityhistory.org/moments-in-disability-history/. Accessed February 19, 2024.

Du Bois, W. E. B. (1898). *Economic Co-operation Among Negro Americans*. Atlanta, GA: Atlanta University Press.

Fink, L. (2022). *Workingmen's Democracy: The Knights of Labor and American Politics*.

France, D. (2016). *How to Survive a Plague: The Story of How Activists and Scientists Tamed AIDS.* New York: Alfred A. Knopf.

Halkitis, P. (2015). *The AIDS Generation: Stories of Survival and Resilience*. New York: Cambridge University Press.

Hämäläinen, P. (2022). *Indigenous Continent: The Epic Contest for North America*. New York: Liveright Publishing Corporation.

Hartman, T. (2021). *The Hidden History of American Healthcare: Why Sickness Bankrupts You and Makes Others Insanely Rich*. Oakland, CA: Barrett-Koehler Publishers, Inc.

Hine, D., Hine, W. C., & Harrold, S., (2010). *The African-American Odyssey*. Upper Saddle River, NJ: Pearson Prentice Hall.

hooks, bell (2014). *Feminist Theory: From Margin to Center* (3rd ed.). New York: Routledge.

Jones, M. S. (2020). *Vanguard: How Black Women Broke Barriers, Won the Vote, and Insisted on Equality for All.* New York: Basic Books Hachette Book Group.

King, M. L. (1991). *A Testament of Hope: The Essential Writings and Speeches Martin Luther King, Jr.* New York: HarperOne.

Liu, Y. L. (2018, May 22). For Asian Immigrants, Cooperatives Came from the Home Country. www.yesmagazine.org/democracy/2018/05/22/for-asian-immigrants-cooperatives-came-from-the-home-country. Accessed January 15, 2023.

Maddox, T. (2018). More than Auxiliary: Caribbean Women and Social Organizations in the Interwar Period. *Caribbean Review of Gender Studies*, 12, 67–94.

National Coalition Against Censorship. Top 10 Banned Books that Changed the Face of Black History.https://ncac.org/news/blog/top-10-banned-books-that-changed-the-face-of-black-history. Accessed February 1, 2023.

Nembhard, J. (2014). *Collective Courage: A History of African American Cooperative Economic Thought and Practice.* University Park, PA: The Pennsylvania State University Press.

Ortiz, P. (2018). *An African American and Latinx History of the United States.* Boston, MA: Beacon Press.

Pfaelzer, J. (2007). *Driven Out: The Forgotten War Against Chinese Americans.* Berkeley, CA: University of California Press.

Pycior, J. L. (2014). *Democratic Renewal and the Mutual Legacy of US Mexicans.* College Station, TX: Texas A&M University Press.

Rivera, J. A. (1984). Mutual Aid Societies in the Hispanic Southwest: Alternative Sources of Community Empowerment. University of New Mexico UNM Digital Repository. https://digitalrepository.unm.edu/shri_publications/34/. Accessed September 10, 2022.

Robinson, C. R. (2000). *Black Marxism: The Making of the Black Radical Tradition.* Chapel Hill, NC and London: University of North Carolina Press.

Rodriguez, M. D. R. (2001). Mexico's Vision of Manifest Destiny During the 1847 War. *Journal of Popular Culture*, 35(2), 41–50.

Singh, N. P. (2017). *Race and America's Long War.* Oakland, CA: University of California Press.

Steele, M. (2020). *Indigenous Resilience.* https://papers.ssrn.com/sol3/papers.cfm?abstract_id=3357805. Accessed December 1, 2022.

Still, W. (2019). *The Underground Railroad Records* (Ed. Q. T. Mills). New York: Modern Library.

Thompson, B. (2002). Multiracial Feminism: Recasting the Chronology of Second Wave Feminism. *Feminist Studies*, 28(2), 337–360.

Wang, C. (2020, April 13). The Chinese Hospital in San Francisco Is Still One-of-a-Kind. www.atlasobscura.com/articles/chinese-blamed-19th-century-epidemics. Accessed January 15, 2023.

Wolff, R. (2014). *Democracy at Work: A Cure for Capitalism.* Chicago, IL: Haymarket Books.

Wright, C. (2014). *Workers Cooperatives and Revolution History and Possibilities in the United States.* Bradenton, FL: BookLocker.com.

Zinn, M. B. & Dill, B. T. (1996). Theorizing Difference from Multiracial Feminism. *Feminist Studies*, 22(1), 321–331.

Chapter 3

Luminaries of Group and Community Psychology

Robin McCoy Brooks

The term mutual aid is generally associated with activist and social justice movements; however, in the last century forerunners emerged in group and community psychology that were also influenced by these principles. These visionaries developed their research from clinical experiences within groups and communities, long before the field of psychosocial studies emerged at the turn of the 21st century. The luminaries of psychosocial and mutual aid–influenced psychology are Jacob Levy Moreno, the originator of the term group psychotherapy and founder of psychodrama, sociometry, and sociodrama; Ignacio Martín-Baró, the founder of liberation psychology in the Global South; and William Schwartz, who, among other social workers introduced the concept and term mutual aid into the field of group social work.

These distinct theories and methods emphasize empowering person and group within their environment, the centrality of relationships, social justice, and mutual aid approaches. Each movement arose in response to what was found to be missing from mainstream psychology and their critiques remain relevant today (Moreno, 1953; Schwartz, 1959; Martín-Baró, 1994). As such, their work contributed to a body of knowledge that is recognized today as psychosocial studies (Frosh, 2015).

As discussed in our book's introductory chapter, psychosocial studies is a relatively new approach to social and psychological research that perceives the individual as both social and psychological and constituted by many conscious and unconscious formations (Frosh, 2003). Applied psychoanalysis (or depth psychology) is a term used to describe how psychosocial theorists have extrapolated theoretical aspects of depth psychology to explore unconscious processes in group and community relations, institutions, cultures, and historical eras (Hook, 2008; Wu, 2013; Frosh, 2015; Watkins, 2019; Saban, 2020).[1]

Psychosocial psychoanalytic studies draw on the works of Eric Fromm, Franz Fanon, Ignacio Martín-Baró, Kimberlé Crenshaw, Gloria Anzaldúa, Jessica Benjamin, Michael Foucault, Jacques Lacan, Judith Butler, and Slavoj Žižek, to name a few. While the founder of liberation psychology, Ignacio Martín-Baró, is happily included in this list, other luminaries of group/community research and

DOI: 10.4324/9781003386339-5

practice are not. These include J. L. Moreno and William Schwartz, among other social workers, as discussed below.

In this chapter, we highlight the works of Moreno, Martín-Baró, and Schwartz, whose basic assumptions about healing have contributed to how each of us have carried their wisdom forward, including what has led us to the birth of this book.

Jacob Levy Moreno: Founder of the Group Psychotherapy Movement

Jacob Levy Moreno (1989–1974) was a Romanian-born American psychiatrist most known for his pioneering work in group psychotherapy, psychodrama, and sociometry. He is generally considered to be a founder of the group psycho-therapy movement itself, and was the first to formally introduce the actual terms "group psychotherapy" and "group therapy" in 1932 at the annual conference of the American Psychiatric Association in Philadelphia.[2] Additionally, Moreno organized several of the first American and international societies of group therapists now known as the American Society of Group Psychotherapy and Psychodrama (ASGPP) and the International Association of Group Psychother-apy (IAGP). This abbreviated biographical list of Moreno's pioneering achieve-ments must also include his contribution to the field of social network analysis through the science of sociometry, which focuses on a quantitative evaluation of an individual's positioning or role in a particular community or group (J. D. Moreno, 2014).

The libidinal engine behind Moreno's prolific corpus can be found in its phil-osophical underpinnings. Moreno's cosmology was a comprehensive system of theory and technique that grew from a philosophy of life that incorporated the biological, psychological, social, and metaphysical dimensions of experience, seen as an interacting organic whole. He believed that every person contained an "autonomous healing center" (the Godhead), proclaiming that "each of us is a genius" (J. L. Moreno, 2019, p. 4). In this fundamentally egalitarian view, we are perceived as not only capable of self-healing but as co-responsible for contributing to the healing of each other in moving towards a world we can fall in love with.[3]

A community, Moreno (1953, p. xv) claimed, had the potential to heal itself from collective subjugation if it embraced three principles. The first was that spontaneity-creativity was a propelling force within each of us, and if tapped collectively could transform a group, individual, and society into a new dimen-sion of functionality and purpose. Expressions of care ("love") and mutual aid ("mutual sharing") were crucial to a group's cohesion and a foundation for a "super-dynamic" community if "newer techniques" were applied (Ibid.). All of Moreno's methods were cultivated to mobilize the propelling force of crea-tivity that, when accessed, can individuate a community towards its greater purpose.[4]

Early Conceptions of Group Therapy

Moreno initially conceived of group therapy as a treatment for those most oppressed in society, and gravitated towards refugees, prisoners, and the severely mentally ill (Nolte, 2014). Keenly aware of the oppressive larger socio-economic and political environment following World War I, Moreno was motivated to experiment with public theater as a vehicle for the expression of social freedom. He experimented on children in public parks, for example, where he extended *play* into storytelling in action. Children would play the role of God and other characters in these stories, in what today is called Playback Theater.[5] While Moreno intended to use theater to mobilize social change, he observed that earlier, when working with sex workers, for example, the participation was therapeutic for both the audience and those enacting the scenes (J. L. Moreno, 2019).

Moreno's philosophy of communal healing in action can be illustrated by his own charming account of an incident in 1913, where the *idea of group psychotherapy* was first developed (J. L. Moreno, 1953, p. xxviii). Moreno was on a street in Vienna and began talking to a young woman who had just smiled at him. As they began to talk, a policeman arrested her and took her to the police station. Moreno was inspired to follow them and waited until she was released, whereupon he befriended her. He learned that she had been arrested because she was a sex worker and was dressed "too provocatively" during the daytime. Soliciting customers was only allowed after dusk.

He was then inspired to organize a collective of sex workers into something like a labor union, so that they, too, could become self-respecting and respected. Moreno initiated these efforts by organizing groups to meet several times a week in the workers' homes, accompanied by a specialist in venereal disease and a local journalist. He described how the initial outcomes of these meetings were pragmatic and involved finding a lawyer, seeking medical care, and collecting minimal dues so that each person could rely on savings for emergencies. Eventually, Moreno began to notice that something different was happening on a psychological level as each person was becoming "a therapeutic agent for each other" (J. L. Moreno, 1953, p. xxx). This opened his mind to the very real possibilities of group therapy.

Moreno and Freud

Moreno did not disavow individual psychology but believed that the *individual and society co-created* itself with a whole range of outcomes. If we wanted to maximize the well-being of a group, collective, or society, he claimed, we needed to work with the inter-relational dynamics within the group while recognizing how the individual's inter-psychic dynamics are also at play (J. L. Moreno, 1953). His philosophical system was in part a critique of Freud and Jung's psychoanalytic, highly individualistic stance that was gaining stature in the newly developing fields of psychiatry and psychology, in Europe and the United States, at the turn of the 20th century. This critique can be encapsulated by an encounter he likely had with Freud at the University of Vienna in 1912. Moreno had just attended a lecture of Freud's that included an interpretation of a telepathic dream. Following the lecture, Moreno recalled commenting to Freud:

> Dr. Freud, I start where you leave off. You meet people in the artificial setting of your office. I meet them on the street and in their homes, in their natural surroundings. You analyzed their dreams; I try to give them courage to dream again.
>
> (J. L. Moreno et al., 1964, pp. 16–17)

Moreno's comment suggests a sharp critique of both the urbane quality of Freud's psychotherapy and its adherence to the self-contained individual, a critique that remains relevant for how much of psychology is practiced today.[6] Moreno's words to Freud indicate how his methods and ideas also straddled the split between the treatment of the isolated mind (as in talking therapy) and the treatment of the group's collective conscious and unconscious realities.

For Moreno, the treatment of the group's conscious and unconscious also contributed to the individual's psychological formation, although his theories of both were distinct from psychoanalytic discourse.[7] His broader vision embraced healing at a societal level, later articulated in 1934 thus: "A truly therapeutic procedure cannot have less an objective than the whole of mankind" (J. L. Moreno, 1953, p. 3).

Psychodrama and the Psychosocial

Psychodrama remains one of Moreno's signature methods. It grew from his early social experiments in Vienna, and later clinical experiences in the United States. Theory evolved from clinical experience. Moreno offered a variety of definitions of psychodrama throughout his works, incorporating elements of religion, sociology, psychology, theater, and socio-political realities. Psychodrama is a science that explores the "truth" by dramatic methods, dealing with "inter-personal relations and private worlds" (J. L. Moreno, 1953, p. 81); it is a "theology" (J. L. Moreno, 1921), a "dramatic art form" (J. L. Moreno, 1924), a "socio-political system" (J. L. Moreno, 1953), a "method of psychotherapy" (J. L. Moreno, 1946), and a "philosophy of life" (J. L. Moreno, 1955).

For our purposes, Peter Felix Kellerman may offer a more comprehensive definition of psychodrama in *Focus on Psychodrama: The Therapeutic Aspects of Psychodrama*:

> Psychodrama is a form of psychotherapy in which clients are encouraged to continue and complete their actions through dramatization, role playing, and dramatic self-presentation. Both verbal and nonverbal communications are

utilized. A number of scenes are enacted, depicted as memories of specific happenings in the past, unfinished situations, inner dramas, fantasies, reams, preparations for future risk-taking situations, or unrehearsed expressions of mental states in the here and now. These scenes either approximate real-life situations or are externalizations of inner mental processes. If required, other roles may be taken by group members or by inanimate objects. Many techniques are employed, such as role reversal, the double, the mirror, concretizations, maximizing and soliloquy. Usually the phases of warm up, action, working through, closure and sharing can be identified.

(Kellerman, 1992, p. 20)

Psychodrama is thus an experiential approach that moves a group process forward through various modes of individual and collective action. Rather than maintaining a focus on the personal dynamics of the individual alone, the group must be treated as a whole. Moreno was concerned with working with the sociodynamics of the entire group, which would include the personal dynamics of the individuals in the group, as well as the interrelationships and interactions between the group members. Everybody has something to teach the group about itself, and everyone can teach each other.

Setting the Stage: Psychodrama and Sociodrama

Group process work of any kind is messy, and I would be negligent if I failed to describe the underbelly of group process work. Whenever we, or any of us, gather in a room, there are divisive undercurrents of *othering*—those split-off shards of psyche that become activated in a collective field. Each of us carries a shadow (in Jungian parlance) around with us, a trace of our wounds, a psychical limp that is *not known* (unconscious) and resisted. These shadow dynamics shape subjectivity and intersubjectivity throughout the various stages of group development. The unconscious makes itself known in dreams, fantasies, regressive splitting, projecting, scapegoating, blurts, moods, verbal and non-verbal expressions, affect, repression of desire, insecurity, isolation, acting out, resilience fatigue, co-dependency, gallows humor, internalized invisibility, and spirals of hopelessness, merely to name a few.

Psychodrama is protagonist centered while also working with the group as a whole. By this I mean that the whole group is engaged in the enactment, by witnessing the psychodrama as an audience member and/or by joining the protagonist on the stage by playing various roles in support of an unfolding process.

Sociodrama, on the other hand, is an action method that focuses *the whole group* on a particular theme. In the words of Moreno, "The true subject of a sociodrama is the group" (J. L. Moreno, 1953, p. 87). Sociodrama investigates the intergroup relations and collective ideologies that shape these relations and exposes us to our critically unheld narratives (unconscious) about ourselves that have been enabled by cultural norms (Ulon & Brooks, 2018).[8] While a collective theme usually emerges, a sociodrama, in my practice does not totalize the individual's personal experience into a collective "we." While we may share similarities, such as "having AIDS," "mother loss," "being adopted," "war trauma," for example, there remains a space for what is irreducible to universals, in the space of collective pain.[9] A sociodrama can stand on its own or emerge alongside a psychodrama. Or a psychodrama can turn into a sociodrama, as I illustrate below.

The three phases of either a psychodrama or sociodrama process are: Warm-up, the Enactment, and Sharing. In the warm-up, we begin by creating an environment that conveys safety, encourages self-revelation with others, promotes a spirit of generosity, and begins to establish a mutual aid ethos. A mutual aid ethos is socially contextualized in how leaders and group members treat each other. Mutual aid is the well spring through which cohesion can be established so that the individual and group as a whole may move into a transformative process. The basic function of the warm-up phase is to build a cohesive foundation of care, which is a prerequisite for in-depth individual and group explorations.

From the onset, we ask the group members to participate in creating a large circle, leaving an empty space in the center (usually) that will be the "stage." Everybody places themselves on the perimeter of the stage. Furniture is moved around collaboratively and stragglers are welcomed. Once our space is created, if this is the first session of a longer retreat, I introduce myself (and co-leaders, if applicable), briefly starting with my name and a brief but personal comment about what is present for me. Others are encouraged to do the same, tapping their neighbor on the (R or L) shoulder when finished. We create a confidentiality agreement that everybody agrees with. Session time frame (bathroom, next meal, etc.) and general guidelines are discussed. Anyone who has physical or other medical needs is attended to.

Once group norms are discussed, we move into pre-action-based explorations to warm group members up to their singular purpose for being there. Lusijah usually starts with guided (hypnotic) imagery that directs the individual inward in search of a resource (inner guide, image, word) to access during the session or retreat. There are similarities between guided imagery and the self-guided practice of active imagination discovered by Jung, discussed in Chapter 9. John Mosher and Dale Buchanan often used animal spirit cards that group members selected from the deck. Each card represented an archetypal (universal) theme and often held personal significance to the participants' warm up process.[10]

Any of the pre-warm-up activities can then be enacted or shared and may lead to a variety of sociometric explorations (dyads, sociograms, spectrograms, sculpts, etc.) that are designed (often *in situ*) to enhance group connectivity and build group cohesion.[11] Our purpose is to tap into the animating creative force within the individual that reveals a singular healing purpose that is heightened in co-engagement with group members. In a psychodrama, the selection of a protagonist is the outcome of the warm-up phase. For a sociodrama, the moment the group moves into action, circumambulating around a common theme, signals the enactment phase.

As the group moves into the *Enactment phase*, themes begin to emerge that eventually clarify the collective purpose of a particular session. A protagonist emerges by bringing their inner (self to self) and outer (self to other) dimensions to the stage. This process is facilitated and honed through a variety of action techniques. In a sociodrama, many individuals carry aspects of a theme that becomes concretized as an entire group.

The *Sharing or integration phase* closes the session at the completion of the enactment. The group regathers and literally shares their personal experience of playing the role or as a witness of the enactment. Each of us comes home to ourselves, in other words, having engaged directly or indirectly with a collective experience that may be psycho-activating. Psycho-activating experiences shake us to our core, often revealing a singular truth that occurs through an encounter with another and others. Group leaders typically join in the sharing process. Advice is *not* given, as this is a time for individual group members to express their personal identifications and embodied responses to the work.

Illustration of a Psychodrama and Sociodrama

I recall an unforgettable and powerful psychodrama that turned into a socio-drama during the second day of a retreat session on the Oregon Coast. It was 1992, and the AIDS death rate was horrifyingly undeterred by medical treatments available at that time. Twenty-eight participants attended, most of whom were living with an HIV or AIDS diagnosis. After the warm-up period, I asked the group who would like to be a protagonist. We were in the third day of our retreat and the group, to my mind, was already warmed up for action. I was standing in the middle of a large stage area surrounded by a large circle of group members. A group member named Jim (disguised name) stood up and slowly joined me. His body spasmed with emotion as he approached, unable to speak. I asked if I could put my hand on his back and he nodded, falling into me.

Once the first wave of his feeling subsided, I suggested we walk slowly together around the center of the spacious room (stage). "How can we help you today," I asked, walking slowly together while waiting for Jim to find his words. After several circles, Jim suddenly blurted out the name "Jacob." "Tell us who Jacob is, Jim?" I asked. He lowered his head as waves of sorrow passed through his body as we continued to unsteadily walk. "May I hold your hand," I asked— holding my hand out to him. "Yes," he whispered, grabbing on to my whole arm for dear life. "He is … *was* my partner," he answered with a shudder. "He is dead." We continued to walk as Jim slowly blew out staccato-like phrases, spraying out his words with the conviction of a mother giving birth.

Oddly, I recall envisioning at this moment whales expelling air from their blowholes when they surface, breathing out before they inhale and then returning to the deep. Jim was indeed opening to the depths of his grief. I had a sense that he needed to know that group members were also accompanying him and said, "Look into their faces, as we walk ... I want you to see that you are not alone today." He looked into the compassionate faces of the audience, one at a time—many of which were tearing up as well. His body seemed to steady some.

Jim suddenly stopped walking for a minute, looking down, and then blurted out several more names of friends who also had died of AIDS. At this moment, my whole body shuddered. How many deaths was he carrying, I wondered? I scanned the stricken faces of the group. How many deaths are *they also holding* ... and further ... *how many deaths to AIDS are we all holding*? I then grasped that we were approaching a timeless altered state of inexplicable horror that had been hanging in the air like raw sewage all along.[12] In a flash, I intuited that the protagonist and audience were forming a kind of solidarity through the shared experience of *massive loss*. The intolerable weight of so many deaths was impossible to bear alone. I understood that we needed to create a space that stretched out and slowed down the experience of exponential loss so that we could honor our dead together.

With this in mind, I pivoted into a sociodrama format, in support of the protagonist and the group as a whole. I asked the audience to raise their hand if they, too, had lost loved ones to AIDS. Almost everyone had. I told Jim that his work was opening a grief in others, saying that I wanted to more actively include the group at this point. He concurred, eagerly. I then asked the audience to: "Please walk with us if you have lost up to five friends and lovers." Several members joined us. "Tell us the names of your loved ones, one at a time," I said, as we walked somberly around the room. I continued in this manner, asking audience members to join the procession if they had sequentially lost 10 loved ones, then 20, and so on until the last person to join the walking body had *lost over 100 loved ones to AIDS*. At some point, names could not be remembered, so I asked participants to picture the faces of the dead, which they did, and we continued walking, now holding each other, sweating, weeping, blowing noses, or wiping snot on sleeves ... as memories emptied out into the light of day.

As our group energy depleted, I concluded the action, entering into the sharing phase. Everybody returned to their seats, outside of the stage. I noticed that the circle was reconfiguring as individuals formed new alliances, placing themselves accordingly. Jim was no longer seated alone. His head was resting on someone's shoulder on his left side, and his feet were held by the person on his right side. I asked the group to share their individual experience one at a time, when or if they were ready. Poignant stories were shared about those who had died as Kleenex boxes were passed around.

Grief can also open us to outrageous laughter, another form of release. Humorous stories about our dead also flooded into the room. For many, this was the first time they could openly grieve their losses with others who were sympathetic. Social repression, the denial of the traumatic effects of AIDS, and the chronicity of loss fatigue contributed to these circumstances. The psychodrama had transformed into a memorial ceremony for our collective dead. What had been repressed in everyday life was now, shamelessly, revealed. Love lost was love found again, and honored.

Psychodrama Today

Following his death in 1974, Moreno's third wife—Zerka Moreno—would continue, extend, and clarify J. L.'s corpus.[13] Crucially, in 1975, Zerka also solidified its efficacy by establishing *The American Board of Examiners in Sociometry, Psychodrama and Group Psychotherapy.* This organization was created to establish and monitor the standards for certification around the world, and continues to this day. Moreno's prolific contributions to the field of group psychotherapy remain generally marginalized by mainstream psychology, along with other group approaches. His work, by his own admission, was "controversial" because it deviated from the mainstream psychiatry and psychology of the time (J. L. Moreno, 1953, p. cviii; Gershoni, 2009, in Giacomucci, 2021, p. 34). However, the broader effects of his personality affected the degree to which his corpus remained outside mainstream academia. This phenomena extends to what has been called the "Credentialing Industrial Complex" for mental health workers (Giacomucci, 2021, p. 44). Jonathan Moreno (J. L.'s and Zerka's son) claims that his father's commitment to the *metaphysical* or mystical underpinnings of his core philosophy and his "bombastic personal style and megalomania" were "too much for regular members of the academic community to bear" (J. D. Moreno, 2014, p. 144).[14]

Since Moreno's death in 1974, sociometry and psychodrama continues to point to an ambiguous future (Giacomucci, 2021). The turn towards a medicalized model of mental health treatment focusing on evidence-based methodologies with individuals and reliance on third party payment systems has contributed to the decline of interest in group methodologies in general. Psychodrama's theory and group-as-a-whole approach is based on the practical and metaphysical (psycho-spiritual, unconscious, etc.) dimensions of experiential change, spontaneity/creativity, and community practice, making it difficult to conduct quantitative research. That, in turn, often renders psychodrama ineligible for review as an evidence-based practice by the American Psychological Association (Giacomucci, 2021, p. 44).

Outside of the US, however, psychodrama enjoys a growing popularity. It is practiced in the Global American South, Australia New Zealand, Europe, Turkey, Israel, Taiwan, and China, to name a few.[15] Other countries have designated psychodrama as a scientifically efficacious practice and have established graduate degree programs in both sociometry and psychodrama (Orkibi & Feniger-Schaal, 2019, in Giacomucci, 2021, p. 44). Scott Giacomucci (2021, p. 45) offers a poignant observation about the countries that do have rigorous psychodrama communities. These communities, he notes, "place significant value on community, inter-personal relations and expression."[16] This he contrasts with the values of individualized-focused treatment within the medicalized model that dominates American mental healthcare today.

In the last decade, however, there has been an uptick in psychodrama research.[17] It was as late as 2018 when the American Psychological Association formally recognized group psychology and group psychotherapy as a *specialty*, creating new possibilities for its inclusion in educational and certifying programs (Whittingham et al., 2021).

Liberation Psychology Movement and Ignacio Martín-Baró

In 1989, Project Quest was formed amidst the *spiritus mundi* of HIV/AIDS activism as same-sex relationships became legal, for the first time, in Denmark. The struggle of decolonization heightened under the government of state president F. W. de Klerk, as he began to dismantle the apartheid system in South Africa.[18] On November 7, 1989, the Berlin Wall was destroyed, signifying the dissolution of Soviet rule in Central and Eastern Europe. Seven days later, amidst this revolutionary *zeitgeist*, Ignacio Martín-Baró (1942–1989), the founder of the liberation psychology movement in the Global South, was brutally murdered, along with five Jesuit brothers, their housekeeper, and her teenage daughter. U.S.-*trained* troops of the elite Atláctl Battalion shot them in the head in a courtyard of the Universidad Centroamericana José Simeón Cañas (UCA) in the Republic of El Salvador. The tragedy occurred within a maelstrom of massacres, tortures, rapes, disappearances, and imprisonments of countless Salvadorian people during the Salvadorian Civil War from 1979–1992. The UN could only *estimate* that more than 75,000 people, including children, were murdered in what some scholars claim was a genocidal rampage.[19]

While the UCA massacre drew renewed international geo-political concerns regarding crimes against humanity, it also invigorated interest in Martín-Baró's specific contributions to the field of psychology in the United States. Martín-Baró was a Spanish-born psychologist who had trained at the University of Chicago. His legacy includes a number of articles clarifying the liberatory mission of South American psychology through a rigorous critique of psychology as a whole. It was posthumously published in English.

Roots in Liberation Epistemology

As with all schools of psychology, liberation psychology emerged from a wider historical geo-political and religious context. Liberation *epistemology* was born from the recognition of the needs of oppressed peoples in general. Its origins were in South America. Gustavo Gutiérrez, a Peruvian philosopher,

Dominican priest, and Catholic theologian is generally considered to be the "father" of liberation *theology*. His seminal text, entitled *A Theology of Liberation* (1971/1988) was both a theological and a practical call for believers to take responsibility for their biblical commitment to the poor through action. Gutiérrez extended the narrow considerations of theological discourse of the time to the actual material and economic conditions of the poor in South America. The work inaugurated South American *liberation theology* in the Catholic Church in the 1950s and 1960s. Outside of the Catholic Church, the central tenets of liberation theology have inspired the emergence of Black, Jewish, Islamic, Jewish, Latina, and feminist liberation theologies, to name a few (Watkins, 2019, p. 85).

Greatly influenced by Gutiérrez, philosopher and pedagogist Paulo Freire (1921–1997) would famously develop the notion of consciousness (*conscientizacaó*) in a seminal text entitled *Pedagogy of the Oppressed* (Freire, 1970/2018). Consciousness for Freire was not a passive process. Rather, it involved the struggle to become fully human amidst systemic disempowering relations, socio-political transactions, and ideological conditions that coalesce with self-identity (Freire, 1970/2018, pp. 43–69).Consciousness "requires a profound rebirth," stated Freire, a kind of existential rupture that throws us to our knees (Freire, 1970/2018, p. 61). Perhaps we encounter a catastrophic reality (psychosocial, political, eco) that is incomprehensibly evocative ... and we cannot turn away (Brooks, 2022).

Engaging such a rupture has the potential to reveal a singular "truth" that radically alters one's perspective. It can require us to take on a new form of existence. French philosopher Alain Badiou (2003) describes such an "event" of truth as an exposure to "radical ... love," such as the love we can have for our neighbor. We are opened to a chaotic urge for life that requires us to work *tirelessly with love*, even in the face of unspeakable atrocity.

Martín-Baró: Conscientizacaó, Mental Health, and the Applied Ethics of Responsibility

Simultaneously, the work of Martinique-born psychiatrist Frantz Fanon would influence both Freire and Martín-Baró. Fanon delineated the psychopathology of colonization and highlighted the importance of *de*colonization for the liberation of oppressed people, especially throughout the African diaspora.[20] He advanced what at the time was an extremely radical perspective by elucidating the visceral effects white domination has on Black identity. Fanon's project included autoethnographic studies conducted among the Black middle class in the French Caribbean. Leaning on the work of Fanon (and others), Martín-Baró would further argue that psychology needed to consider the mental health of the poor, and with it socio-political or "psychosocial" forms of oppression. So, for Martín-Baró, psychological outreach would extend into the service of facilitating social change amidst the repressive effects of "psycho-social trauma" experienced by communities that had been subjugated through political violence, war, and poverty (Freire, 1994, pp. 124, 135). In this sense, Martín-Baró introduced the term and phenomena of "psycho-social" trauma that psychosocial studies would extend into the 21st century.

Martín-Baró was also inspired by the tenets of liberation theology, especially Freire's notion of critical consciousness. By developing the work of critical awareness of one's socio/political reality, he sought to de-idealogize dehumanizing narratives and empower individuals to narrate *their own reality* (Martín-Baró, 1994, p. 41). The passion he held for his *"pueblo"* of Salvadorian *"campesinos"* penetrated his writings, especially his unwavering belief in a future of justice and peace that *each person could bring about themselves in the face of its impossibility.* In this way, mental health and social reform are not just connected; they are in many ways the same thing. As Martín-Baró cogently stated:

> If the foundation for a people's mental health lies in the existence of humanizing relationships, of collective ties within which and through which the personal humanity of each individual is acknowledged and in which no one's reality is denied, then the building of a new society, or at least a better and more just society, is not only an economic and political problem; it is also essentially a mental health problem … we cannot separate mental health from the social order
>
> (Martín-Baró, 1994, pp. 120–121)

This statement encapsulates the philosophical underpinnings of Martín-Baró's psyche-social ontology, founded on an *applied* ethics of responsibility held by the individual, the collective, and the psychologist. A society that values humanizing relationships is a predicate for mental health. Recall the conclusions of social scientists Christakis and Fowler (2011), discussed in Chapter 1, that shed further light on what is humanizing. Christakis and Fowler found that expressions of altruism, reciprocity, and emotional care enhance our propensity for reciprocity and cooperation (aspects of mutual aid) and our capacity to build socially altruistic social networks.

While Martín-Baró's immediate focus was to help his parishioners break away from soul-crushing fatalism, he also envisioned that his work was relevant for other oppressed peoples (anywhere) who were likewise yoked to the sidelines of (their particular) histories. His vision was to help them to "break the social structures that rigidly served the interests of the few" (Martín-Baró, 1994, pp. 219–220).

Thus, Martín-Baró identified three urgent tasks that are necessary to nourish the process of acquiring critical *conscientizacaó*, extending the work of Freire, from which a community can mobilize on their own behalf.

First, we must acquire a critical understanding of ourselves and the socio-political existance that we are embedded in, including the recovery of historical memory (Martín-Baró, 1994, p. 30). This involves recovering not only the sense of our personal identities, but also remembering our traditions, cultures, and ancestral heritages that we can carry forward in the service of liberation and freedom from socio-cultural induced fatalism by taking hold of our own fate (Martín-Baró, 1994, pp. 30, 41, 217).

Second, we must de-ideologize ("decode") our everyday experiences against the prevailing discourses ("the lie") that deny, ignore, or disguise the essential aspects of personal reality, *and* we must eliminate those belief systems that sustain paralyzing fatalism (Martín-Baró, 1994, pp. 31, 40, 113). This is accomplished by an *active dialectical process with others* with whom we may *identify our own reality (truth)* (Ibid.).

Finally, we must "utilize the virtues of our peoples" (Martín-Baró, 1994, p. 31). These virtues live in the social structures (traditions, everyday practices, ancestorial heritage, and belief systems) that have contributed to the people's survival, solidarity, and resilience through generations (Martín-Baró, 1994, p. 83).[21]

The Rehabilitation of Psychology Through Social Responsibility

Martín-Baró argued that the role of the psychologist in South America (and everywhere else) was to accept "our social responsibility" *and* regenerate the field of psychology as a whole into a psychology of liberation that functions in response to a people's *real demands* (Martín-Baró, 1994, pp. 33–46). Let us take a breath as we take in the power of his vision for psychology. For whom, he asks, does psychology work?

> The critical questions that psychology must formulate with regard to its activity, and, it follows, with regard to the role it is carrying out in society, should not be centered on where the work is done, but rather on by whom; nor should it be looking at how something is done, so much as for whose benefit.
>
> (Martín-Baró, 1994, p. 45)

In other words, the location, status, and technique one uses is secondary to the *real and urgent needs of the recipient*, whoever the psychologist is. Thus, a liberatory psychologist must first critique the dominating contemporary knowledge systems, *measuring them against* the real problems of those who are marginalized by society, within one's place in history (Martín-Baró, 1994, p. 121). We must "place ourselves" at their "historical lookout point" and denude ourselves from the role of the expert (the one who knows) so that the *dialogic process of truth finding* is "found (by the person and group) and not made" (Martín-Baró, 1994, pp. 27, 45).

Social psychologist Mary Watkins (2019) describes this process as *psycho-social accompaniment*, practiced with individuals and groups who have been abandoned and left to fend for themselves in unimaginable psychological and material situations. This means that the mental health worker becomes a co-participant with, a mirror to, a convener, a deep listener, questioner, witness, and facilitator of the group process. In this way, individuals can make their own sense of the world and discover the breadth of their own capacities and possibilities— in short, a prelude to social change.

Central to Martín-Baró's criticism of mainstream psychology was its Western Eurocentric emphasis on the treatment of the autonomous individual who is seen a-historically and therefore not rooted in any socio-political-cultural historical context (Martín-Baró, 1994, pp. 91–92). He opposed universalizing theories about the individual, systems, and cultures that view each as "discrete universes of meaning" without regard to its relationship to society at large or the environment or cultural history (Martín-Baró, 1994, pp. 92–93). Groups, individuals, or systems may be characterized in stereotypes to justify the systemic oppression of a popular majority, reflected in uncritically held psychological theory and practices prevalent in mainstream psychology (Martín-Baró, 1994, pp. 84–86). The prevalent practice in mainstream Western psychology, which frequently passes without critique, is to characterize persons, groups, or systems as stereotypes.[22] This is reflected, Martín-Baró argued, in biased categorizations of whole peoples, such as the "shiftless Latino", the "lazy Indian," the North American "Protestant ethic," and the "Latin American Catholic ethic" (Martín-Baró, 1994, pp. 198–211).

Lastly, Martín-Baró challenged the academic framework that privileges quantitative research–based theory and praxis *over* lived experience—or qualitative forms of research (Martín-Baró, 1994, pp. 27–28, 98, 184). Instead, he envisioned the thickening potential for building liberatory communities comprised of safe and constructed spaces that awaken people and groups to their individual agentic power. Agency opens to the flexibility to create new collective identities, moving towards shared life-giving goals. This is realized only by breaking away from superstructural constrictions that quash self-knowledge and agency (Martín-Baró, 1994, pp. 217–220).

The brilliance of Martín-Baró's critique is that *he challenges each of us to apply the principles of critical consciousness to ourselves and with each other in relation to the psychological theories and practices of our time.* This examination can become a force of transformation towards a more socially engaged and inclusive psychology (one aimed at social freedom) rather than perpetuating a blind conformity to the social arrangements and theories that lead to consequences such as violence, dehumanization, marginalization, exclusion, material, eco and emotional impoverishment, classism, and greed. We return to this critique and uplifting account of contemporary liberatory projects that are challenging psychology's status quo in Part III of this book.

The Mutual Aid Group Movement in Social Work

Roots of Community-Based Social Work, Social Reform, and Mutual Aid

Social work with groups and the relationship to social reform is generally traced to the turn of the 20th century in the United States. At this time, mutual self-help (as we have seen in Chapter 2) was proliferated across ethnicities, genders, classes, cultures, and communities by the formation of labor unions, societies, and fraternal associations, largely in response to the displacement caused by industrialization, structural racism, the massive influx of immigrants, World War I, the "Spanish" flu, and the impending Great Depression. Mutual aid–based social work with groups would emerge and extend some of the basic tenets of the settlement group model amidst competing interests. Social work was a developing profession that would achieve a full professional status in the 1920s and 1930s.

The settlement movement model of social reform (1880s–1920s) was formally introduced in the United States by Jane Addams, who learned about the system while traveling to England. On her return, Addams and Ellen Gates Starr founded the Hull House in 1889, in Chicago, Illinois. At this time, women were excluded from visible leadership roles throughout most levels of government and business (Kraus, 1980).Contrary to these oppressive social arrangements, women were pioneers in the founding and maintenance of the settlement movement as they determined the structure, ethics, and responsibilities of what was becoming a social welfare movement. Some settlement houses were funded by religious organizations, such as the Christodora Settlement House, located in the slums of New York City's Lower East Side. Its founders, Christina Isobel MacColl and Sarah Carson, were inspired by the social activism of Jane Addams and Lillian Wald, but they would go on to combine their religious motivations with the principles of the settlement idea (Hopkins, 2011). Chicago's Hull House, in contrast, was a secular project because their leaders did not want to discourage their diverse immigrant neighbors from participating.

A central goal of the movement was to bridge the class divide by bringing volunteer middle-class settlement workers (often women) into shared living situations with the poor. Their intention was to co-facilitate improvements in living conditions with the local residents within the community. At the same time, social reforms were introduced in education, sanitation, recreation, female and child labor, and housing, opposing discrimination (Lee & Swenson, 2005). Addams introduced her workers to the idea of *accompanying* (recall Mary Watkins, above) the residents in everyday life, so that both social worker and resident could learn about, and teach, each other. They "must be content to live quietly side by side with their neighbors until they grow into a sense of relationship and mutual interests" (Adams, 1961, p. 98). Towards this aim, the settlement workers organized small groups to establish reciprocal resident-to-resident *and* worker-to-resident relationships (Woodroofe, 1962).

In alignment, John Dewey and his cohorts frequented the settlements and introduced leisure-time group activities. They had the idea that facilitating open sharing and mutual discourse within recreation activitieswould further individual and group development (Lindeman, 1980, pp. 77–82).[23] The timeless practice of mutual relationality, peer group self-help, democratic ideals, and social reform was incorporated into the early social work movement. These pioneers would lay down a foundation for later waves of developing group practice within the diversifying fields of social work, psychology, psychiatry, and psychoanalysis.

The Discipline of Social Work Faces an Identity Crisis

Group work became formally associated with social work practice in 1935 (Giacomucci, 2021, p. 19). Group workers and social organizers attempted to conceptualize their differing theories and methods in a series of special sessions held at the National Conference of Social Work in 1935 and 1939. These efforts would result in the formation of two organizations: the National Association for the Study of Group Work in 1935 (later renamed the American Association of Group Work [AAGW]) and the Association for the Study of Community Organization in 1939 (Giacomucci, 2021).

As group work was establishing itself, the discipline of social work as a whole was facing its own identity crisis amidst the dominating discourse of psychoanalysis. Psychoanalysis focused on the intrapsychic dynamics of individual suffering, within a one-on-one (casework) clinical setting. In a move to remain relevant, the social work field would operationalize its model of mental health treatment by adopting an individualized, intrapsychic understanding of trauma and adjusting its treatment focus *away* from "the problems of the poor" towards the middle and upper classes (Ehrenreich, 2014, pp. 60, 75, in Giacomucci, 2021. pp. 20–21).

In 1969, the Council on Social Work Education (CSWE) changed its accreditation standards for social work education by structurally eliminating the specialization areas of casework, group work, and community organization. The intent was to promote a more holistic and *generalist approach* to social work practice (Simon & Kilbane, 2014, in Giacomucci, 2021 p. 19). The change in orientation towards a generalist approach in social work education would align with emerging psychiatric (medicalized) models of mental illness and behavioral, or evidence-based, practices (EBP) that dominate mental healthcare today (Hyde, 2013, p. 43).

Mental illness, in other words, was, and continues to be, understood through the lens of individual pathology, disregarding broader environmental contexts (Conrad, 2007, pp. 7–8). The reconfiguring of social work into a generalized practice would institutionally degrade the value of group perspectives, including mutual aid–oriented groups (although not referred to as mutual aid then) and social reform justice motivations, known as social justice today. This initiative is often critiqued as the catalyst for the subsequent 40-year decline of group work in social work education (Knight, 2017, in Giacomucci, 2021, p. 20; Giacomucci, 2021, pp. 18–19).

To this day, social work education programs offer little specialized group work training. Students are often thrown into practicum settings without adequate preparation (Knight, 2017, p. 20). Because group training is generally not institutionally valued, the message conveyed to practitioners is that they don't need it or can figure it out on their own. Amidst this backdrop, group work would nevertheless tirelessly continue to be a major component of social work practice within a wide range of settings, including inpatient and outpatient residential programs, hospitals, mental health clinics, and private practice into the 21st century.

William Schwartz Coins the Term Mutual Aid in Social Work with Groups

Social worker William Schwartz first coined the term "mutual aid" with groups in 1961. As Schwartz's work developed, he would radically shift the source of healing from the group leader to the members themselves (Schwartz, 1977). His definition of a "mutual aid" group is as follows:

> … the group is an enterprise in mutual aid, an alliance of individuals who need each other, in varying degrees, to work on certain common problems. The important fact is that this is a helping system in which the clients need each other as well as the worker. This need to use each other, to create not one but many helping relationships, is a vital ingredient of the group process and constitutes a common need over and above the specific tasks for which the group was formed.
>
> (Schwartz, 1977, p. 19)

In his view, the group leader provides a mediating function in order to activate the mutual aid function, already present in the group, as a means of overcoming many obstacles that will inevitably challenge its effectiveness. The mediator works in the *group as a whole system* in order to activate the inter-dependencies group members have on each other. Helping relationships are born and developed, and exponential resources are thus created and shared (Steinberg, 2003, pp. 36–37).

Schwartz's vision of mutual communalism was a corrective against the sociopolitical forces that supported the ideological myths of the self-made person (man), discussed in Chapter 1. He was concerned about the dehumanizing effects of a superindustrial society, including patterns of segregation, and the inability of transient and disorganized people to pool their interests and mobilize together on their own behalf.[24] The cult of rugged individualism reinforces the belief that we are responsible for ourselves, and that our interdependency on each other is a weakness. This is supported by neo-liberal policies and corporate practices today (Quart, 2023). In this sense, Schwartz was a social activist, as well as a scholar and clinician whose theories and practices were developed and refined amidst a minority groundswell of other like-minded social workers.

Contemporary Social Worker Approaches to Mutual Aid Groups

Contemporary social worker streams have expanded the theory and practice of mutual aid–based group work today by emphasizing the goal of social agency and action (Gitterman & Shulman, 2005; Glassman, 2009; Steinberg, 2014). While it is beyond the scope of this chapter to fully summarize these contributions, I have compiled a list of core principles of mutual aid group approaches developed in contemporary social worker research:

1 Mutual aid groups embrace health-centered (strength based, recovery focused) perspectives, in contrast to pathology-oriented perspectives. The foundational belief is that each individual and group have unique positive resources and resilience from which they may heal and heal each other from the basis of a shared humanity (Steinberg, 2010, 2014; Saleebey, 2012; Hyde, 2013; Gitterman & Knight, 2016).

2 Mutual aid groups promote healing from adverse (trauma) experience, thereby opening the individual and group to transformative possibilities for the individuation of self and group. This may alter existential belief systems, spiritual dimensions, relational enhancement, and agency in the group and one's world (Calhoun and Tedeschi, 2014; Wu et al., 2019; Giacomucci, 2021, pp. 169–171).

3 Mutual aid groups may integrate non-deliberative and deliberative practices, dependent on the purpose, kind of group, and psychological orientation of the group leader.

4 Mutual aid group process is facilitated through the lens of the group as a whole, in contrast to working with one individual at a time. Group cohesion is facilitated by attending to the intergroup dynamics in a group process where differences and similarities are revealed, shared themes emerge, and inter-dependencies can be formed. The expectation is that group members will use each other to meet their needs (Northen & Kurland, 2001; Steinberg, 2003).

5 "Mutual aid is both a process and a result. As a process, mutual aid is what group members do together to be helpful. As a result, it is what group members experience from having interacted with others in a particular way" (Steinberg, 2014, p. 21).

6   Group leaders oversee the creation and maintenance of a mutual aid system from an ethos they practice, teach, and promote, which Schultz (1961) referred to as "lending a vision." Group leaders retain a light hierarchical position, while authority is shared with the group on decisions that affect the group as a whole.

7   Engaging in a mutual aid process is empowering and increases a sense of self-efficacy so that members are able to engage in purposeful mutual aid and build relational skills and mastery in other environments (Shulman & Gitterman, 2005; Knight & Gitterman, 2014).

8   There are various models of mutual aid group development in the social work literature. Urania Glassman (2009, pp. 197–226) describes eight stages that cogently and creatively grasp the themes of a group's development: Stage one: *Criteria for assessing member* (ego capacity and sense of self-capacity to engage in a democratic process); Stage two: *We are not in charge* (approach to difference, biases, sameness, belonging and authority, fantasies about vulnerability emerge); Stage three: *We are in charge* (engages with struggles and/or resistances regarding inclusion, exclusion, uncertainty about place in group, and capacity of leadership); Stage four: *Sanctuary* (freely engages in mutual aid with others, can work through differences, leader is no longer only idealized); Stage five: *This isn't good anymore* (fluctuating difficulty in sustaining purpose in the face of challenge and fearful of deepening intimacy with self and others); Stage six: *We're okay and able* (able to change, take risks, face fear or failure); and Stage seven: *Just a little longer* (actualizing purpose requires taking stock of growth in the face of ambivalence and broadening options such as leaving the group) (Glassman, 2009, pp. 197–226).

9   There are a variety of group settings where mutual aid approaches can be practiced, including short-term groups, single-session groups, open-ended groups, and structured groups. Specific agendas, time constraints, fluctuating membership, psychosocial features, and setting (community, institution, clinic, private practice, clinician training/supervision/education) place unique dilemmas for group leaders using a mutual aid approach (Glassman, 2009).

10 Mutual aid groups are inclusive. This means the facilitator must be familiar with the role of intersectional oppression in group members' lives based on race, cultural practices and belief systems, social class, gender, biological identity, age, ability, religion, national origin, and immigrant status, to name a few (French et al., 2020).

11 The values underlying mutual aid practices include building trust and relationships with group and community members through reciprocity, collaboration, creativity, flexibility in structure, cooperation, connection and authentic relating, shared humanity (inclusivity), community-driven care, the redistribution of resources, and generativity and action in responsive to needs (Littman, et al. 2022).

We have a better sense of the competencies required when working with mutual aid–oriented groups and communities from this pithy compilation. The next section elaborates two categories of group practice that occupy the field of social work today.

Deliberative and Non-deliberative Approaches to Social Work Group Practice

Several modes of group practice, and their supporting theories, have evolved in the social work field that Norma Lang describes in two categories: *deliberative* and *non-deliberative* (Lang, 2016). A *deliberative* model to group practice is characterized as verbal, didactic, linear (step by step), and cognitively directed towards a reasoned, problem-solving purpose. Many academic classes, training modules, and clinical supervision groups are organized in a deliberative model, as are psycho-educational groups and cognitive behavioral based therapy (CBT) groups, for example. Many research projects are dominated by deliberative processes determining the guidelines for how scholarly research is composed and published. Conative problem-solving work in a group setting is analytic, verbally descriptive, explorative, and elaborates the data of life experience. While affect is a feature of both processes, in the deliberative model participants are removed from the embodied sense of experience in order to scrutinize it (Lang, 2016, p. 103).

Lang describes the *non-deliberative* approach to group practice as providing avenues for member expression that exceeds discussion-based approaches. The non-deliberative sphere of art, play, action, and analogue is designed to be experiential, process-oriented, spontaneous, intuitive, creative, *verbal and non-verbal* (Lang, 2016, pp. 100, 102, 103, 107). *Discourse*, in the words of philosopher Emmanuel Levinas, is "not contained to language alone but what is *communicated and received by the other*, including silence" (Levinas, 1969, p. 195; my emphasis). Discourse, Levinas elaborates, "is the experience of something absolutely foreign, a *pure* knowledge or experience" (Levinas, 1969, p. 73; my emphasis), "probably [beginning] through traumatisms or groupings to which one does not even know how to give a verbal form: a separation, a violent scene, a sudden consciousness of the monotony of time" (Levinas, 1985, p. 21).

Levinas introduces us to the metaphysical components of expression that when considered opens the individual and group to another dimension of exploration. In psychodynamic terms, we are talking about the enigmatic traces of the unconscious—our complexes, what is blocked from awareness, such as our biases, as well as access to the fullness of our life force. These enigmatic traces of being emerge through the body into our awareness if there is a therapeutic space to receive and explore them. The psychodrama/sociodrama illustrated in the first section of this chapter is an example of a non-deliberative group process. The protagonist was accompanied by the group as a whole into what became a co-created space where our dead could be collectively honored and mourned. Later, in the sharing phase, we moved into a deliberative mode where each member reflected (narrativized) what they experienced during the enactment.

Experiential process groups offer alternative spaces, providing access to new ways of knowing by exploring and communicating emergent realities. Other modes of exploration include action methods, play, art, art therapy, music, dance, dramatics, simulation, role play, rehearsal, poetry, journaling, psychodramatic methodologies, psychedelic medicine healing practices, hypnotic visualization techniques, Jungian dream interpretation, Jungian active imagination, and Jungian arts-based research. Jungian scholar Susan Rowland and artist Joel Weishaus have extended the arts-based research methodology to Jungian psychology (Rowland & Weishaus, 2021). In Rowland's words, Jungian arts-based research "opens therapy and research to the whole world by accessing knowledge through creative collaboration with the wisdom of centuries materialized in other traditions and the unknown psyche" (Rowland, 2023, p. 437). In Chapter 9, I elaborate on the potential of Jungian arts-based research that is both clinical and research oriented for the field of psychology today.

While the categories of non-deliberative and deliberative modalities may appear to be mutually exclusive, Lang is keen to underscore how these two discrete ways of understanding and exploring life experience *can work together* towards diverse therapeutic purposes. In an earlier paper, Lang argued that working with non-verbal and/or actional modalities mobilized agency with "socially unskilled persons in groups" (Lang, 2010, pp. 172–181). Our experience in the formation of the Quest community supports Lang's claim, as many of the participants had never been in individual or group therapy and were experiencing various forms of collective trauma. Body work (of all sorts) is crucial when language is impaired, words don't come, and preverbal, unconscious, or unformed expressions emerge in an individual or a group. Eventually, using language to express one's reality, self-knowledge, or *conscientizacaó* within a social context supports individual and collective agentic power, as elaborated by Martín-Baró. Indeed, using both methodologies respects the many ways individual minds and bodies comprehend experience and the many aims for forming a group.

Today, the deliberative approach to group work is the dominant method utilized in the social work arena (Giacomucci, 2021, p. 21). However, the integration of non-deliberative mutual aid–based group practices among social workers is gaining traction. This is noted by the 2019 symposium on non-deliberative approaches by the International Association for Social Work with Groups (Sullivan et al., 2019). Furthermore, a movement of social workers is actively engaging in dialogue with the theories and practices of psychodrama, especially in the area of mutual aid group theory and practice (Gershoni, 2009; Skolnik, 2018; Giacomucci & Stone, 2019; Giacomucci & Marquit, 2020).

Scott Giacomucci is one of the prominent theorists and practitioners of experiential group work and is both a social worker and Trainer, Practitioner, and

Educator (TEP) of psychodrama, sociometry, and group psychotherapy. In a recent work (2021) entitled *Social Work, Sociometry, and Psychodrama*, Giacomucci advocates for the inclusion of action methods and other non-deliberative approaches to group social work, including detailed accounts of both traditions, such as how they overlap from a philosophical, theoretical, and clinical basis.

Closing Thoughts

We have seen how the distinct group movements of psychodrama, liberation psychology, and social worker group practice overlap in their emphasis on egalitarianism, placing social justice at the center of training, the centrality of relationships, strength and resiliency, mutual aid practices, healing and transformation through self-knowledge, group/community development, and socio-political action. Another shared basic assumption views the psychological dynamics of the individual as inseparable from the socio/political realm. Thus, the liberation of the individual and their social mileau is inextricably tied to the transformation of society.

Part I of this book has provided the socio-historical context for the rest of the book. Part II, entitled "The Quest Story," describes the psychological, relational, political, socio-cultural, and creative climate that spawned the emergence of a hybrid mental health and mutual aid clinic in 1989. We describe how the community was formed amidst the AIDS crisis, our roles, and how we developed our group ethos, methodologies, and theories in quickly moving situations. We also reflect on the pitfalls of mutual aid group practice and our errors. This part of the book is an articulation of what we learned then about the transformative power that ordinary people can have when they mobilize together to create systems of care in the shadow of socio-political systems that don't.

Notes

1 See the Mary Watkins book entitled *Mutual Accompaniment and the Creation of the Commons* (2019). Watkins states in her introduction: "My focus … [is] an intentional move away from models based on individualism and unidirectional helping to those that acknowledge our inherent interdependence and potential mutuality. I turn away from expertism and toward mutual, dialogical, participatory, and horizontal relations" (p. 1).

2 These include Joseph Pratt, Trigant Burrow, and the advent of social workers with groups (discussed below), to name a few. For other historical accounts of the etiology of the term and practice of group psychotherapy, see J. L. Moreno (1945); Renouvier (1958); Z. T. Moreno (1966); Giacomucci (2021), p. 32.

3 Moreno described such a cosmic person as "an individual who is close to all beings, not really apart from them but with them and within them, involved with all men, animals and plants. He believes himself to be a part of the universe and not a member of a family or clan. Everyone is a brother or partner to him, – he does not make any distinction between rich and poor, black or white, man or woman. Everyone is his friend, and he wants to help everybody" (J. L. Moreno, 2019, p. 339).

4 Leaning on Moreno, Robin has elsewhere referred to this psyche-social dynamic as "trans-subjectivity" from which the individual may move from personal concern to social responsiveness and action towards manifesting a collective aim. See *Psychoanalysis, Catastrophe & Social Action* (2022).

5 See Jonathan Fox, Ph.D., Trainer, Practitioner, and Educator of psychodrama, sociometry and group psychotherapy (TEP) and co-founder of Playback Theater in *Beyond Theatre: A Playback Theatre Memoir* (2019, Tusitala Publishing). Playback Theater is widely practiced internationally. Fox is also the author of many other books.

6 Personal conversation with Daniel Masler, August 22, 2023.

7 Robin picks up this thought in Chapter 9 in a discussion of how C. G. Jung and Moreno differed and overlapped in how they theorized what the unconscious is and how it manifests and is treated.

8 Siyat Ulon and I co-facilitated a sociodrama in Cape Town, South Africa, at a professional conference sponsored by the International Association for Jungian Studies in 2018. Our paper (Ulon & Brooks, 2018) describes how we introduced an action method into an academic setting and the collective themes that emerged.

9 Today there are a number of authors who work with and write about the theory and practice of collective and intergenerational trauma in experiential, mutual aid–based groups from different psychological traditions. See Mollica (2006); Kellerman (2007); Leveton (2010); Nieto (2010); Hudgins & Toscani (2013); Figusch (2014); Linklater (2014); Steinberg (2014); Van Der Kolk (2014); Dayton (2016); Hübl (2020); Giacomucci (2021); Ordóñez (2021), to name only a few.

10 John Mosher, TEP, died of COVID-19 two years ago. We co-led weekly psychodrama groups for 30 years. John was a charismatic and gifted trainer, author, and psychotherapist, co-leading many Quest psychodrama AIDS men's retreats with Dale Buchanan in the later AIDS era. Dale was my TEP on-site examiner in the 1990s as I was finishing my TEP training during an AIDS retreat on Mt Hood. Dale and John were sociometric stars in the broader psychodrama community for many years. Dale recently retired from long-standing leadership on the Board of Examiners, having influenced the training processes of thousands of psychodramatists for decades. One of Dale's favorite sayings was "Never pass by an open pocket." He was not advancing pick-pocketing but encouraging us to attend to the synchronistic opportunities that fate and "tele" provide us. Tele is a loaded concept put forth by Moreno that I develop further in Chapter 9 in relation to transference. In brief, tele is a "function of group cohesiveness, reciprocity of relationships, communication, and shared experiences" (J. L. Moreno, 1960, p. 17). Moreno defines tele as "insight into and appreciation of, and feeling for, the actual makeup of the other person" (Ibid.). Tele operates through our social desires, our choices, and our behavior in relationships (p. 18).

11 It is beyond the scope of this book to adequately describe the various kinds of action techniques that a certified or trained psychodramatist has lodged in their back pocket. We direct the interested reader to a few classic texts on the subject. Start with Scott Giacomucci's 2021 book entitled *Social Work, Sociometry, and Psychodrama Experimental Approaches for Group Therapists*. Also, Sternberg and Garcia (1989), Blatner (2000), and Kellerman (2007).

12 When a society or community cannot mourn their dead because of socio-cultural-induced repression, such as in this case unexpressed grief, it remains in the collective shadow.

13 See Moreno, Z., Horvatin, T., & Schreiber, E. (Eds.) (2015) *The Quintessential Zerka: Writings by Zerka Toeman on Psychodrama, Sociometry and Group Psychotherapy.*

14 One can see parallels for the declining popularity of C. G. Jung's analytical psychology.

15 Noted in the *American Board of Examiners in Psychodrama, Sociometry and Group Psychotherapy* directory for Certified Practitioners of Psychodrama (CP) and

Trainers, Educators, and Practitioners (TEP). This site contains relevant information about the certification process as well. See: https://psychodramacertification.org/

16 The research approach we adopt in this book, for example, is qualitative, ethnographic, and arts-based research. Qualitative research is the dominant approach recognized by the American Psychological Association and mainstream journals, publishers, and academia.

17 Ulon & Brooks (2018), Skolnik (2018), Orkibi & Feniger-Schaal (2019), and Giacomucci & Marquit (2020), to name a few.

18 See anthropologist Vincent Crapanzano's study of late-apartheid South Africa, entitled *Waiting: The Whites of South Africa* (1985). Crapanzano describes a predominating mode of collective waiting experienced by those who dominate (empowered white people) in opposition to apartheid. "For most whites," he states, "waiting is compounded by fear; for most blacks, however great their despair, waiting is illuminated by hope, by a belief that time is on their side. For coloured's and Asians, there is both fear and hope in waiting" (in Brooks, 2022, p. 141).

19 See the "Report on the UN Truth Commission on El Salvador," www.derechos.org/nizkor/salvador/informes/truth.html, March 29 1992. Scholars differ on whether the atrocities that occurred during the Civil War could be considered as genocide. See: https://impakter.com/el-salvadors-forgotten-genocide-40-years-later/ by Victor Aguilar Pereira. The murder of intellectual elites, or sophiacide, such as Martín-Baró and many of his colleagues is only one of the defining categories of genocide.

20 See Fanon, F. (1963). *The Wretched of the Earth*. New York: Grove Press.

21 *Māori* activist and academic Linda Tuhiwai Smith highlights in her influential work entitled *Decolonizing Methods* how the question of knowledge in the context of "decolonization of methods" is crucial. She argues that knowledge institutions need to examine/critique the roles that knowledge, knowledge production, and knowledge hierarchies play in social transformation (Smith, 2012, p. xii). Tuhiwai Smith introduces us to the decoloniality movement embraced by philosophers, cultural theorists, anthropologists, social scientists, activists, psychologists, and feminists radicalized by dehumanizing physical and psychical effects of colonization. Decoloniality is a way to habilitate knowledge that has been subjugated by the forces of modernity, settler-colonialism, and "racial capitalism" (Brooks, 2022).

22 I am grateful to Daniel Masler for this insight, personal conversation 9/10/23.

23 A recreational arm named Team Quest within the Project Quest community was created and led by community members. See Chapter 6 for a lengthy discussion of how Team Quest projects evolved and were reported in the local newspapers, including a documentary about Team Quest mountain climbing (produced by Greg Fowler and Christopher Carloss) that aired on public television. Part II, Chapters 4 and 5 include other accounts of Team Quest activities as each of us participated.

24 On this, Schwartz stated: "The call for a new individualism is an attempt to find a solution to the loss of human dignity; but in its plea for a new assertion of self, it proposes the one against the many and seeks the sources of freedom in man's liberation from his fellows rather than in the combined effort of men to control their environment" (Schwartz, 1959, p. 27).

References

Adams, J. (1961). *Twenty Years at Hull House*. New York: Signet.

American Board of Examiners in Psychodrama, Sociodrama and Group Psychotherapy. (n.d.). https://psychodramacertification.org/. Accessed April 2, 2022.

Badiou, A. (2003). *Saint Paul: The Foundation of Universalism*. Stanford, CA: Stanford University Press.

Blatner, A. (2000). *Foundations of Psychodrama: History, Theory, and Practice*. New York: Springer Publishing Company.

Brooks, R. M. (2022). *Psychoanalysis, Catastrophe & Social Change*. New York and London: Routledge.

Calhoun, L. G. & Tedeschi, R. G. (Eds.) (2014). *Handbook of Posttraumatic Growth: Research and Practice*. New York: Routledge.

Christakis, N. & Fowler, J. (2011). *Connected: How Your Friends' Friends' Friends' Affect Everything You Feel, Think, and Do*. New York: Little, Brown Spark.

Conrad, P. (2007). *The Medicalization of Society*. Baltimore, MD: John Hopkins Press.

Crapanzano, V. (1985). *Waiting: The Whites of South Africa*. New York: Random House.

Dayton, T. (2016). *NeuroPsychodrama in the Treatment of Relational Trauma: A Strength-Based Experiential Model for Healing PTSD*. Deerfield Beach, FL: Health Communications Inc.

Ehrenreich, J. H. (2014). *The Altruistic Imagination: A History of Social Work and Social Policy in the United States*. New York: Cornell University Press.

Fanon, F. (1963). *The Wretched of the Earth*. New York: Grove Press.

Figusch, Z. (2014). *The JL Moreno Memorial Photo Album*. London: lulu.com.

Fox, J. (2019). *Beyond Theater: A Playback Theatre Memoir*. New Paltz, NY: Tusitala Publishing.

Freire, P. (1970/2018). *Pedagogy of the Oppressed*. New York: Bloomsbury Academic.

Freire, P. (1994). *Pedagogy of the Oppressed*. Cambridge, MA: Harvard University Press.

French, B. H., Lewis, J. A., Mosley, D. V., Adames, H. Y., Chavez-Dueñas, N. Y., Chen, G. A., & Neville, H. A. (2020). Toward a Psychological Framework of Radical Healing in Communities of Color. *The Counseling Psychologist*, 53(4), 14–46.

Frosh, S. (2003). Psychosocial Studies and Psychology: Is a Critical Approach Emerging? *Human Relations*, 56, 1547–1567.

Frosh, S. (2015). *Psychosocial Imaginaries: Perspectives on Temporality, Subjectivities and Activism* (S. Frosh, Ed.). New York: Palgrave Macmillan.

Gershoni, J. (2009). Bringing Psychodrama to the Main Stage in Group Psychotherapy. *Group*, 33(4), 297–308.

Giacomucci, S. (2021). *Social Work, Sociometry, and Psychodrama: Experiential Approaches for Group Therapists, Community Leaders, and Social Workers*. Singapore: Springer.

Giacomucci, S. & Marquit, J. (2020). The Effectiveness of Trauma-Focused Psychodrama in the Treatment of PTSD in Inpatient Substance Abuse Treatment. *Frontiers in Psychology*, 11, 896.

Giacomucci, S. & Stone, A. M. (2019). Being in Two Places at Once: Renegotiating Traumatic Experience Through the Surplus Reality of Psychodrama. *Social Work with Groups*, 42(3), 184–196.

Gitterman, A. & Knight, C. (2016). Promoting Resilience Through Social Work Practice with Groups: Implications for the Practice and Field Curricula. *Journal of Social Work Education*, 53(4), 448–461.

Gitterman, A. & Shulman, L. (2005). *Mutual Aid: A Buffer Against Risk. Mutual Aid Groups, Vulnerable & Resilient Populations, and the Life Cycle*. New York: Columbia University Press.

Glassman, U. (2009). *Group Work: A Humanistic and Skills Building Approach*. London: Sage Sourcebooks for Human Services.

Gutiérrez, G. (1971/1988). *A Theology of Liberation*. New York: Orbis Books.

Hook, D. (2008). *Six Moments in Lacan*. London and New York: Routledge.

Hopkins, J. (2011). The Sacred and the Secular in Christodora Settlement House 1897–1929. *Social Welfare History Project*. https://socialwelfare.library.vcu.edu/settlement-houses/the-sacred-and-the-secular-in-christodora-settlement-house-1897-1939/. Accessed February 10, 2023.

Hübl, T. (2020). *Healing Collective Trauma: A Process for Integrating Our Intergenerational and Cultural Wounds*. Boulder, CO: Sounds True.

Hudgins, M. K. & Toscani, F. (2013). *Healing World Trauma with the Therapeutic Spiral Model: Stories from the Frontlines*. London: Jessica Kingsley Publishers.

Hyde, B. (2013). Mutual Aid Group Work: Social Work Leading the Way to Recovery-Focused Mental Health. *Social Work with Groups*, 36(1), 43–58.

Kellerman, P. F. (1992). *Focus on Psychodrama: The Therapeutic Aspects of Psychodrama*. London: Jessica Kingsley.

Kellerman, P. F. (2007). *Sociodrama and Collective Trauma*. London: Jessica Kingsley Publishers.

Knight, C. (2017). Social Work Students' Experiences with Group Work in the Field Practicum. *Journal of Teaching in Social Work*, 37(2), 138–155.

Knight, C. & Gitterman, A. (2014). Group Work with Bereaved Individuals: The Power of Mutual Aid. *Social Work*, 59(1), 5–12.

Kraus, H. P. (1980). *The Settlement House Movement in New York City, 1886–1914*. New York: Arno Press.

Lang, N. C. (2010). *Group Work Practice to Advance Social Competence*. New York: Columbia University Press.

Lang, N. C. (2016). Nondeliberative Forms of Practice in Social Work: Artful, Action, Analogic. *Social Work with Groups*, 39(2–3), 97–117.

Lee, J. & Swenson, C. R. (2005). *Mutual Aid: A Buffer Against Risk*. In A. Gitterman & L. Shulman (Eds.), *Mutual Aid Groups, Vulnerable & Resilient Populations, and the Life Cycle*, pp. 573–596. New York: Columbia University Press.

Leveton, E. (2010). *Healing Collective Trauma Using Sociodrama and Drama Therapy*. New York: Springer Publishing Company.

Levinas, E. (1969). *Totality and Infinity*. Pittsburgh, PA: Duquesne University Press.

Levinas, E. (1985). *Ethics and Infinity*. Pittsburgh, PA: Duquesne University Press.

Lindeman, E. C. (1980). Group Work and Democracy – a Philosophical Note. In A. S. Alissi (Ed.), *Perspectives on Social Group Work Practice*, pp. 77–82. New York: Free Press.

Linklater, R. (2014). *Decolonizing Trauma Work: Indigenous Stories and Strategies*. Halifax: Fernwood Publishing.

Littman, D. M., Boyett, M., Bender, K., Dunbar, A. Z., Santarella, M., Becker-Hafnor, T., Saavedra, K., & Milligan, T. (2022). Values and Beliefs Underlying Mutual Aid: An Exploration of Collective Care during the COVID-19 Pandemic. *Society for Social Work and Research*, 13(1), 89–115.

Martín-Baró, I. (1994). *Writings for a Liberation Psychology*. Cambridge, MA: Harvard University Press.

Mollica, R. F. (2006). *Healing Invisible Wounds: Paths to Hope and Recovery in a Violent World*. Orlando, FL: Harcourt, Inc.

Moreno, J. D. (2014). *Impromptu Man: J. L. Moreno and the Origins of Psychodrama, Encounter Culture, and the Social Network*. New York: Bellevue Literary Press.

Moreno, J. L. (1921). *Das Testament des Vaters*. Vienna: Gustav Kiepenheuer Verlag.

Moreno, J. L. (1924). *Das Stegreiftheater*. Berlin: Bustav Kiepenheuer Verlag.

Moreno, J. L. (1945). *Group Psychotherapy: A Symposium*. Beacon, NY: Beacon House Press.

Moreno, J. L. (1946). *Psychodrama* (Vol. 1). New York: Beacon House.

Moreno, J. L. (1953). *Who Shall Survive? Foundations of Sociometry, Group Psychology and Sociodrama*. Beacon, NY: Beacon House Inc.

Moreno, J. L. (1955). The Significance of the Therapeutic Format and the Place of Acting Out in Psychotherapy. *Group Psychotherapy*, 8, 7–19.

Moreno, J. L. (1960). Tele: A Definition. In J. L. Moreno, H. H. Jennings, J. H. Criswell, L. Katz, R. R. Blake, J. S. Mouton, M. E. Bonney, M. L. Northway, C. P. Loomis, C. Proctor, R. Tagiuri, & J. Nehnevajsa (Eds.), *The Sociometry Reader*, pp. 17–18. Glencoe, IL: The Free Press.

Moreno, J. L. (2019). *The Autobiography of a Genius* (E. Schreiber, S. Kelley, & S. Giacomucci, Eds.). United Kingdom: North-West Psychodrama Association.

Moreno, J. L., Moreno, Z. T., & Moreno, J. D. (1964). The First Psychodramatic Family. *Group Psychotherapy*, 16, 203–249.

Moreno, Z. T. (1966). Evolution and Dynamics of the Group Psychotherapy Movement. In J. L. Moreno (Ed.), *The International Handbook of Group Psychotherapy*. London: Peter Owen.

Moreno, Z. T., Horvatin, T., & Schreiber, E. (Eds.) (2015). *The Quintessential Zerka: Writings by Zerka Toeman Moreno on Psychodrama, Sociometry and Group Psychotherapy*. New York: Routledge.

Nieto, L. (2010). Look Behind You: Using Anti-Oppression Models to Inform a Protagonist's Psychodrama. In E. Leveton (Ed.), *Healing Collective Trauma Using Sociodrama and Drama Therapy*, pp. 103–125. New York: Springer Publishing Company.

Nolte, J. (2014). *The Philosophy, Theory, and Methods of J. L. Moreno: The Man Who Tried to Become God*. New York: Routledge.

Northen, H. & Kurland, R. (2001). *Social Work with Groups*. New York: Columbia University Press.

Ordóñez, E. (2021). *Ancestry: The Deep Field of Reality*. Quechelah Publishing.

Orkibi, H. & Feniger-Schaal, R. (2019). Integrative Systematic Review of Psychodrama Psychotherapy Research: Trends and Methodological Implications. *PLoS ONE*, 14(2). https://journals.plos.org/plosone/article?id=10.1371%2Fjournal.pone.0212575.

Pereira, V. A. (2019). El Salvador's Forgotten Genocide: 40 Years Later. https://impakter.com/el-salvadors-forgotten-genocide-40-years-later/. Accessed January 15, 2023.

Quart, A. (2023). *Bootstrapped: Liberating Ourselves from the American Dream*. New York: HarperCollins Publishers.

Renouvier, P. (1958). *The Group Psychotherapy Movement: J. L. Moreno, Its Pioneer and Founder*. Psychodrama and Group Psychotherapy Monographs, No. 33. Beacon, NY: Beacon House.

Rowland, S. (2023). Jungian Arts-Based Research (JARG): What It Is, Why Do It, and How. *Journal of Analytical Psychology*, 68(2), 436–439.

Rowland, S. & Weishaus, J. (2021). *Jungian Arts-Based Research and the Nuclear Enchantment of New Mexico*. New York: Routledge.

Saban, M. (2020). *Simondon and Jung: Rethinking Individuation*. In C. McMillan, R. Main, & D. Henderson (Eds.), *Holism: Possibilities and Problems*, pp. 91–97. London and New York: Routledge.

Saleebey, D. (2012). *The Strengths Perspective in Social Work Practice*. Boston, MA: Pearson Education.

Schwartz, W. (1959). Group Work and the Social Scene. In A. J. Kahn (Ed.), *Issues in American Social Work*, pp. 110–139. New York: Columbia University Press.

Schwartz, W. (1961). The Social Worker in the Group. In R. Pernell & B. Saunders (Eds.), *New Perspectives on Services to Groups: Theory, Organization, Practice*, pp. 17–34. New York: National Association of Social Workers.

Schwartz, W. (1974). The Social Worker in the Group. In R. W. Klenk & R. M. Ryan (Eds.), *The Practice of Social Work*, pp. 208–220. Belmont, CA: Wadsworth.

Schwartz, W. (1977). Social Group Work: The Interactionist Approach. In *The Encyclopedia of Social Work* (Vol. 2). New York: National Association of Social Workers.

Simon, S. & Kilbane, T. (2014). The Current State of Group Work Education in U.S. Graduate Schools of Social Work. *Social Work with Groups*, 37, 243–256.

Skolnik, S. (2018). A Synergistic Union: Group Work Meets Psychodrama. *Social Work With Groups*, 41–42(1–2), 60–73.

Smith, L. T. (2012). *Decolonizing Methodologies: Research and Indigenous Peoples*. London: Zed Books, LTD.

Steinberg, D. M. (2003). The Magic of Mutual Aid. *Social Work With Groups*, 25(1–2), 31–38.

Steinberg, D. M. (2010). Mutual Aid: A Contribution to Best-Practice Social Work. *Social Work With Groups*, 33(1), 53–68.

Steinberg, D. M. (2014). *A Mutual-Aid Model for Social Work with Groups*. New York: Routledge.

Sternberg, P. & Garcia, G. (1989). *Sociodrama: Who's in Your Shoes?* New York: Praeger.

Sullivan, N. E., Sulman, J., & Nosko, A. (2019). Proposal for the IASWG Symposium Invitational in Honor of Norma C. Lang and Nondeliberative Practice Theory. *International Association of Social Work with Groups (IASWG)*. www.iaswg.org/Nondeliberative-Invitational. Accessed February 25, 2023.

Ulon, S. & Brooks, R. M. (2018). Collective Shadows on the Sociodrama Stage. *International Journal of Jungian Studies*, 10(3), 221–236.

Van Der Kolk, B. (2014). *The Body Keeps the Score*. New York: Penguin Books.

Watkins, M. (2019). *Mutual Accompaniment and the Creation of the Commons*. New Haven: Yale University Press.

Whittingham, M., Lefforge, N., & Marmarosh, C. (2021). Group Psychotherapy as a Specialty: An Inconvenient Truth. *Group Psychology and Group Psychotherapy*, 74(2), 60–66.

Woodroofe, K. (1962). *From Charity to Social Work*. London: Routledge and Kegan Paul.

Wu, K. (2013). Can Individual Psychology Explain Social Phenomena? An Appraisal of the Theory of Cultural Complexes. *Psychoanalysis, Culture & Society*, 18, 386–404.

Wu, X., Kaminga, A. C., Dai, W.., Deng, J., Wang, Z., Pan, X., & Liu, A. (2019). The Prevalence of Moderate to High Posttraumatic Growth: A Systemic Review and Meta-Analysis. *Journal of Affective Disorders*, 243, 408–415.

Part II

The Quest Story

Chapter 4

Project Quest's Story

Lusijah Marx

The Roots of Project Quest

Project Quest began one night with a shared dream. There was mystery and magic in learning that someone else, a young man named Lucas Harris, was dreaming the exact same dream I'd just experienced, even details about my life that he did not know. As a therapist specializing in the field of psychoneuroimmunology in the 1980s, I had been leading psychodrama retreats at Mount Hood several times a year. Lucas, a young man living with AIDS, was a participant and volunteer at the time. The dream happened during a psychodrama healing retreat. Psychodrama is a therapy form using action. Instead of just talking about a situation, the scene is reenacted and becomes alive. At a retreat, we share the same living space, build community, and a collective consciousness is created. This atmosphere holds trust. Participants allow their vulnerability to emerge and with a sense of safety, powerful healing work occurs from addressing past trauma, exploring how to be truthful, assertive, or even tender in relationships in the here and now, or imagining one's future. At retreats for people living with AIDS or other illnesses, dramas often focused on gaining some control by acting out charged experiences, such as becoming disabled or dying. This particular retreat in 1988 changed my life. A group of 15, mostly men living with AIDS and a few women with AIDS or cancer, trudged with backpacks up the snowy hill to the cabin we had permission to use for the weekend. The aim was to build a trusting community to support people living as fully as possible, living authentically until death.

Lusana, a woman with breast cancer, did a psychodrama related to her death and how to stay connected to herself and each of her five children through her dying process. Lucas was chosen by Lusana to play the role of her son Ryan, who was seven years old at the time. This drama was raw and powerful. We each shared what came up personally, and all were deeply moved. That night, I had a dream that Lucas and I were co-creating a community-focused healing center where people could receive care with alternative treatments, such as acupuncture, and address lifestyle patterns such as smoking, drugs, diet, and sleep

DOI: 10.4324/9781003386339-7

in innovative ways. The dream indicated changes that Lucas needed to make related to his relationship, as well as personal work that I needed to do in my marriage to heal my heart. I decided I would tell Lucas the part of the dream that was about him, but only his part.

When we talked that morning over breakfast, I was astounded to hear from Lucas that he had the same dream. He even dreamed the part about healing my heart and the situation with my husband that he knew nothing about. This dream, and the willingness to see it as a calling, changed my life. Following the guidance of the dream also changed Lucas's life and death.

Lucas believed that if we had the same dream, it was necessary for us to carry it out. Neither of us had the skills required for creating a center. Lucas had worked as a hairstylist and I as a clinician. We decided to do meditation each day and ask for guidance and clarity. Over the course of that year, after following up on many ideas, Lucas found a lawyer who had written a book on nonprofits to help us accomplish the paperwork to become a 501(c)3 official nonprofit. From our daily meditation process, we had ideas that helped us find practitioners, and we learned about certain healing modalities to incorporate into our center.

As I reflect on who Lucas was to me, I would define him as my soulmate. He was a gay man with AIDS who touched my heart, and with his love and support deepened my trust and commitment to live authentically. The consciousness we shared felt so vulnerable, yet vast. It was like nothing I had ever experienced. Spirituality for me means listening within for wisdom and a special kind of knowing and willingness to follow that guidance. My soulmate Lucas and I believed and trusted our shared dream and guidance to create what became Project Quest. It is now called the Quest Center for Integrative Health in Portland, Oregon, and still exists today, serving thousands of marginalized people. I believe in dreaming big dreams, trusting your inner wisdom, and following it.

Since the age of 21, I have been engaged in a spiritual path called Subud, which is not a religion, as people from different religions and people who do not believe in God are all welcome. It has at its foundation the value of surrender, opening and embracing one's true self. and inner knowing, which is what my story continues to be about. Experiences with Lucas, who was also in Subud, will be an integral part of my story of how Project Quest came to be and my own story of becoming more fully who I am.

There is wisdom within each of us that heals. It often becomes dormant because of our culture, religious dogma, and our families. I reclaimed my ability to trust and follow my inner guidance by spending time with amazing people, mainly gay men during the AIDS pandemic. I experienced a community that valued love, trust, and being true to oneself. It changed my life. There was such rawness in stepping into a marginalized community that was living in the horror of a terrible, unknown illness that caused unsightly lesions, wasting, fever, fatigue, and death. Stepping into this community, initially to complete research for my doctorate, helped me experience the world with a different lens and to know myself.

As a woman in my late 70s now, I look at who I am and who my people are, the ones who have shaped my life and who helped me believe in dreams. I smile as I remember Lucas, who was so very important in my life, and as I recall my own personal healing journey.

I grew up in Iowa, land where the tall corn grows—and where conservatism, including skepticism, literal belief in the Bible, homophobia, and fixed ideas related to health (doctors know everything, patients know very little) abound. My grandfather Frank, a farmer, was from a fundamentalist church that did not believe in pleasure. He believed that music, dancing, and activities that might be pleasurable were "the work of the Devil." He was stern and ready to punish anyone who looked like they might be having fun. My father had given up his career goals, as his choices were limited by Frank. My mother, whose father and three brothers were ministers, was more progressive in her thinking, but in her actions and feelings as a woman had only a small voice.

I had many ideas of what I might like to do with my life, but being a secretary, store clerk, nurse, or teacher were presented as my options. I graduated from a class of 44 students in Johnston, Iowa, and studied nursing at the University of Iowa (where my father had not been allowed to go, as Frank stated it was "a den of iniquity.")

My sister Lorraine, who was ten years older, was an artist and moved to New York City. I spent my college summers with her and was awakened and dazzled by the diversity. My world began to open. Lorraine joined a spiritual movement called Subud, based on a meditation practice done alone or in community. I initially was skeptical and had no interest. However, during my second summer in New York, I saw that her friends in Subud seemed to be happier and had made positive changes. With my interest in how people change, I decided to join during the summer before my senior year in college. I hoped for insight, and never expected that the practice of meditation would affect me in a profound, life-changing way.

Upon my college graduation in 1966, I planned to join the army and go to Vietnam. Though I was against war, I felt as a nurse I could be of service. By now, I was doing meditation daily and had significant nighttime dreams indicating the army would be a negative choice for my life. So I applied for a nursing job in St. Thomas, Virgin Islands. Two weeks before I was to move, I was awakened three mornings in a row with the same powerful dream each time that I needed to work in New York City. Because of my dreams, I moved to New York and worked on a surgical ward with marginalized people. Working on a surgical ward seemed like the best place to develop my skills. While in New York City,

I attended the Subud group and the practice of daily meditation as the guiding force in my life became stronger.

On a surgical ward, I began to see how frequently health issues came from lifestyle patterns and poverty, and how little attention was focused on prevention. Alcoholics with bleeding ulcers and varices, and diabetics with gangrenous feet, were frequent patients and would be back the next year with deteriorating health. While working with surgical patients I met Leo, a surgical resident at New York Hospital, and fell in love. He was in a program through the navy for doctors, and after his first year of residency was required to go to Vietnam. I went with him to Oceanside, California, for his training. I was 24 and he was 28 when we got married and I was pregnant with our first child.

Leo was stationed with the marines on the frontline in Vietnam. He became very sick and was sent back to the USA to a naval hospital in Philadelphia. When he recovered, he was stationed on a submarine base in Groton, Connecticut, where Robert, our first child, was born. Leo had experienced the horrors of war, and as a doctor on the frontlines injured soldiers either died or were airlifted to Saigon. He developed PTSD with nightmares and flashbacks. With his return to civilian life, he could function, as surgical work required an intense focus that kept daytime flashbacks at bay. He completed his military duty on the submarine base in Groton, Connecticut, his residency in surgery in Hartford, and his thoracic surgery in Milwaukee, Wisconsin. He needed a lot of support and I focused on providing that for him while caring for our four children, born between 1969 and 1974. After Vietnam, Leo always struggled with sleep, and I took on the role of leading him through guided imagery/hypnosis nightly so he could function. Over time, with his difficulty sleeping and mood swings he was diagnosed as bipolar in addition to his PTSD. He did not believe in psychotherapy, and though I was passionate about it, he felt it was irrelevant. Keeping him stable required a tremendous amount of my energy.

When I was 31, Oregon became my home. Leo finished his residencies and we drove cross-country to his new job as a heart surgeon in Portland, Oregon. That drive was unforgettable. I was in a station wagon with four children. Robert, my oldest child, was six, and Hilary, my youngest, not quite one and still nursing. Leo was driving a U-Haul and we were beginning our new life. I had never been to Oregon.

Over the next five years, I completed my master's degree in nursing and changed my focus from medical illness and surgery to mental health. This came about from working on a ward in a VA hospital for people with chronic pain. Daily, I witnessed men with chronic pain who had untreated trauma that clearly affected their ability to recover. It became evident to me that working with the mind/body connection was a key component in addressing pain. I learned medical hypnosis and how often the images and experiences that were healing came spontaneously in altered-state work. Living with pain limited people's lives, and loneliness was a major problem, so addressing isolation was key for successful treatment for many folks. Needing more experience in facilitating groups, I signed up for a five-day training focused mainly on psychodrama. The training was experiential, and we explored group members' issues through role play. It was the most powerful personal therapeutic work I had ever experienced. Most of my therapy had been cognitive, while psychodrama included body, mind, heart, spirit, and community.

In this workshop, I met Robin, who had been working towards psychodrama certification, and I was struck by her intuition, creativity, and talent. We developed a deep love and trust for each other through sharing our lives, including uncertainty, losses, and healing experiences. Little did I know that we would be living a drama together and co-facilitating retreats. Neither of us knew that what we were learning would be foundational in building a community with people living with AIDS.

Dissertation Study with AIDS

In 1981 I started graduate school at Pacific University near Portland, Oregon, for a doctorate in psychology. In my experience of the medical model, very little was directed at inspiring people with illness to address the underlying issues that cause disease, often related to a lack of connection and lifestyle. Witnessing the detrimental split between mind and body inspired me to pursue my doctorate. I had seen the importance of people's beliefs and images about health and well-being in determining outcomes. Therefore, when I came to the point of doing research for my dissertation, I decided I would focus on developing specific hypnotic imagery for people living with life-challenging illnesses. This would include imagining changes within one's body and connecting in a positive way with oneself, work that I had been doing in addressing pain, injuries, and illness for years.

Previously, I taught a number of patients to visualize positive internal changes such as imagining the incredible healing process that goes on within one's body after breaking a bone. Together we would create images of the bone mending and function returning. I also worked with patients using imagery that supported change in bodily functions. For example, hypnotic work appeared to help a man get his blood clotting time down to the level needed to have surgery on his eyes and re-experience his joy of reading. I also worked with hemophiliacs to cut their blood product use in half by learning hypnotic/visualization techniques. Being able to empower one's body by believing in its health and healing capacities helped many people change disease patterns. I witnessed people gain a sense of agency in their own healing using guided imagery, and I saw people commit to greater health by envisioning changing lifestyle patterns and addressing diet, exercise, sleep, belonging, meaning, and self-compassion. My dissertation could help build a body of research on wellness-based health care approaches and systems.

During this time, I read a number of books on mind/body medicine to help me formulate my thoughts and my research. Different authors described personal experiences, often after a loved one or they themselves had an illness that broadened their thinking. Being trained in the medical model, I was steeped in a powerful dogma that limited my thoughts. When I read of spontaneous remissions or people's descriptions of medical breakthroughs, I was automatically skeptical, as I was a part of the medical paradigm which does not accept things that happen that cannot be scientifically explained.

I took a trip to Alaska, where I spent time in nature. The spaciousness of the land, glaciers, mountains, old grove forests, and amazing animals awakened a new, fresh perspective. This setting and daily meditation helped me move out of the fixed mindset I had from my medical training. Spending time in nature in a beautiful land led to my awareness changing. I could think and believe with more openness.

I felt a shift, and I could believe there was much more to healing than what I had been taught. The value of the human spirit and an individual's capacity to heal were of little relevance in my medical training. My trip to Alaska and reading and thinking in this spacious environment were invaluable to me as I now questioned the foundations of my training about health, healing, and access to healthcare.

As I look back on that time, I am aware of how important it is to question the status quo—and how limiting it can be when we meet the gatekeepers, and ultimately when we become the gatekeepers, of what is true, how care is given (or not), and who receives it.

It was challenging to be in a rigorous doctoral program, as well as in my marriage. Over time, Leo's struggles with sleep and his reactivity and control had grown more intense. I was questioning many things both professionally and personally. I continued to attend psychodrama retreats where I felt seen and appreciated in a very different way than I felt at home. Given the demands of my family, I was eager to find my target population, do my research, and finish my program. My experience with the gay community had been narrow and my clinical work had focused mostly on people with cancer or chronic pain.

Around this time, the news was broadcasting accounts of gay men getting sick and quickly dying terrible deaths. I was hearing about AIDS, an illness that had no answers and was spreading. Hospitals were fearful of such patients, and healthcare workers wore gloves and masks if they were willing to deal with AIDS patients at all. As I focused on finishing my doctorate, I wanted to continue exploring my deep belief in the "mind/body connection" that had become stronger in Alaska. This seemed like a population that would be ideal for the work I wanted to do. Since there were no effective treatments, if people improved with guided imagery/hypnotic strategies, it would be easier to credit the changes to this mind/body treatment. My training in hypnosis and guided imagery was in depth and I believed in its value. I realized that if my research was to show the benefits that one's images and beliefs have on health, addressing AIDS was the best choice. In 1987, there was no cure and very little hope for people diagnosed with HIV. I was still looking as an outsider at the AIDS crisis, feeling alarmed and experiencing great compassion for those people, but viewing them as "those people," nonetheless. My decision to focus on AIDS for my study came out of practical concerns—not out of my engagement with the community.

I was using hypnotic approaches developed by Carl Simonton, Jeanne Achterberg, and Marty Rossman in my work. The psychoneuroimmunology approaches used were based on creating a hypnotic state and visualizing one's body effectively doing what it needed to be doing to get better, and envisioning a positive future instead of being caught up in the fear of pain and death from illness. I designed a protocol for participants in my study to envision the virus and to imagine that their T-cells could recognize the virus and do their natural function of engulfing and dissolving it. The imagery continued with imagining the thymus developing and releasing strong, vibrant T-cells and visualizing regaining energy and strength to live life fully again.

My protocol had passed the Human Subjects Review, and I was ready to gather participants whom I would see for ten hypnotic therapy sessions. The subjects would draw pictures of what they visualized after each session. I had a small amount of money for getting a P-24 test, which was a rough test used at that time to measure viral activity. This test would be done at the beginning of the study and again after ten hypnotic sessions. The protocol and goals were clear, and I was excited to begin the project. The first barrier and lesson came as I put the word out about the study to obtain volunteers. I had given flyers for recruitment of subjects to various doctors who worked with people with HIV, but no one came. After six weeks, one person, a man named Tom who received a flyer from his doctor about my study, contacted me. He said he was terrified of his illness and its progression and felt willing to try anything. We met and discussed the study, and he decided he wanted to participate. He told others, and by the next day I had 30 people interested. I began to understand that I was engaged with a very different community than I had dealt with in my past clinical work. The vulnerability, stigma, and rawness of living with AIDS had taught those infected to be much more cautious and reluctant to trust anyone not known by their community. When Tom trusted me and believed this approach could be useful, others followed suit.

My own journey to greater consciousness became stronger as I began to do hypnotic work with each individual. I quickly found that the protocol I had carefully developed was way too limiting. In Tom's first session, he said, "I see myself as a little boy in corduroys," and he began to cry. What was coming to the foreground for him was not the imagery of my protocol, but his childhood trauma.

The people in the study were all gay men with HIV. In our sessions, they were continually drawn to early experiences of trauma where they felt abandoned, lost, bullied, abused, and alone. I struggled with a personal dilemma. I wanted to finish my dissertation and get on with my future. Clearly, the protocol I had designed for this study needed more dimensions. I discovered time and time again trauma affecting participants as we shared in the deep inner place where hypnotic work occurs. After much soul-searching, it was apparent to me that I had to approach my committee and change the direction of my research. Each session could contain some of the protocol, but it had to be individualized by what the inner guidance of the person with HIV tapped into, which was almost always related to trauma.

This decision was a hard one. I had been preparing for this study for a year. I knew I might not get my doctorate if I changed the focus from an evidence-based medical approach with a well-defined protocol. After agonizing for a while, I had a spontaneous epiphany about what to do. My participants were men living with fear and the prognosis of a very short life. They deserved a better experience than my conducting a carefully designed protocol to get my degree. The willingness to go to my committee and present a new plan that was personalized came to me. This was a significant change, as there would be no possibility of replicating it. The new plan focused on developing an individualized model for treatment rather than a protocol with a defined script. Miraculously, my committee agreed. I was able to convince them that my ethics would not allow me to ignore the inner wisdom that prompted the imagery, mostly related to trauma, that the men in my study kept experiencing. My committee members became convinced that developing an effective model was more useful to persons living with AIDS, and to my learning as well.

I began to sense that when the subjects in my study listened to their inner guidance as their imagery developed, it was powerful and useful. They became personally engaged and more empowered to better self-care, and to imagine improved outcomes. The more they listened and followed, the more naturally that guidance came. I, too, was finding how effective and important inner guidance was for me. The more I listened and followed, the more I had clarity, trusting myself both personally and professionally.

The process of imagery as a dance that unfolded by the creation and participation of both me, the therapist, and the person with HIV was magical and transformative. It was much more powerful than what either of us alone could have created. Each person in the study would do the hypnotic session and then draw a picture related to their session, as in the original study plan. Their pictures became less passive and had strong, clear, effective imagery of T-cells recognizing and destroying the virus. The drawings also showed a connection to a more authentic and engaged life. On my end, as the hypnotic work continued to unfold, I was deeply touched by the courage and struggles of the lives of these frightened, courageous men. A deep heartfelt connection and love for each person grew. They were no longer the "other," and neither was I.

When I began this study, I did not know that it would lead me to meet beloved people who would change my life, my beliefs, and my way of practice. I began as an outsider doing research with people who were "other." As I met people with AIDS in the study, my heart had to become wider and stronger to experience the love that I would give and receive in a way I had never experienced within the framework of traditionally structured medicine. In this crisis time, we bonded in a meaningful way. As I entered the intimate process of guided imagery, and as the stories of abuse and loss revealed themselves, there was healing for them and for me. Jack, a friend of Tom's, was one of the men in my initial research study. He was a former priest, as was Tom, who had left the Church and become a strong advocate for social justice. His imagery unfolded, containing the loss of his mother in his teenage years and his struggle with Catholicism and his sexuality. As a priest, he came to a crisis of faith, and left the Church. His profound journey to find himself and his truth was moving to me. As our community was emerging, Jack was a natural leader. He brought advocacy and values that sparked those qualities in others. Throughout his life he was a loving father figure to many who needed a strong, kind presence. He was a man who lived fully, and through his words and actions encouraged others to do the same. Jack became a long-term survivor and died from heart disease in his late sixties, cared for and loved by our community as his health declined.

As each of the study subjects attended ten hypnotic sessions, a fuller engagement in life was happening. I witnessed the themes that emerged in individual sessions and sensed that hypnotic work in a group setting might create a pool of creative ideas. As we began to do group work, creativity increased and the imagery collectively became stronger. A community was forming where people shared together and helped each other. When my dissertation ended, it was clear that I was part of the community, and I would not go back to either private practice or work driven by the medical model. Almost all of the men who used guided imagery were deeply engaged in an inner process that felt meaningful. They were addressing areas together related to living and thriving. There was heartfelt commitment in this community that had grown to include hemophiliacs, women, and heterosexual men. I knew this was my community and I could not leave it to return to the world I had come from.

Early Days of Quest

After the shared dream, Lucas and I continued to meet daily to meditate, followed by creating a plan for the day and addressing the needs of our community. Our vision included people feeling safe, and bringing love, care, and tenderness where there was fear. It also included making soup and having nourishing food available. People who were sick needed to have support and help with chores.

We finally were an official nonprofit and had to have a board of directors. Not really understanding the functioning of a nonprofit board, I invited four medical doctors along with Jack to be board members. At our first official board meeting, one of the research doctors from Legacy Hospital made this comment: "It is clear by your choice of us as board members you plan to do tight research and will need our help to design and implement your research plans." Jack and I looked at each other, aware that was not our plan at all. Instead, we intended to explore with every person who needed help how to find a path towards the greatest wellness possible. It was clear that having a loving supportive community for grounding and maintaining connection had to be part of our mission. Doctors, with no engagement in the actual community itself, could not be the ones to develop our mission. A board of mainly doctors created a power hierarchy that would not support the spirit of our work.

We searched for clarity for the next board. Clarity came. Our community of people living with AIDS were already volunteers supporting our infrastructure, as we had no money to pay staff. They were answering phones, talking to people who were interested in services, and organizing help for those who were sick. These were the people who cared about our mission and were finding renewed energy in involvement. Our next board was made up of volunteers. Brian, a man living with AIDS, became the first chairperson of our board of directors. He came up with our official name, "Project Quest," because he saw healing as a "Quest" that leads to vibrant health and a healing path for all who participate. The name was unanimously liked by the board and our community and became official for our nonprofit organization.

In our daily work, Jack took on fiscal responsibility along with being the person that everyone would go to with practical issues. Lucas was young, handsome, irreverent, and witty, yet deeply spiritual, loving, and sincere. He was a visionary, a dreamer who inspired, and a natural leader. David showed up every day to do the chores, and Brian answered phone calls and did outreach. We sensed the value of a "soft" hierarchy where different people took on responsibility and there was room for fresh input and leadership in different ways.

It was clear that with a wasting disease that had many people struggling with fatigue, we needed to address cooking and eating. Infectious disease doctors were encouraging people to eat anything with calories such as pizza, ice cream, and cookies. We created a program, in conjunction with natural food stores donating nutritious food, which included learning how to select food and cook it. Our cooking was followed by a community dinner where each person was welcomed and supported in finding a sense of belonging. Dinners began with a circle of sharing. Learning the nutritional value of foods that promote health and increased energy was our aim. We would have special days of making healthy dishes and soups to give to those who were sick and to freeze for future use at times of low energy. Quest even had a garden for a time. Sharing a sense of power and participation often led to inspired healing wisdom. In many experiences we felt the intuitive knowledge of the members of our community in conjunction with professionals. Working together was innovative, inclusive, and magical.

In groups, the guidance became stronger for most people and new ideas and friendships blossomed. There was a natural way of showing up with love, compassion, and care. Groups helped individuals identify the need for self-care, to speak up and express feelings and to find their own rhythm for active engagement. This "magic" in a time that held so much fear and death drew many people, and we organically became a community-based program. We moved from being a few people receiving services to address the epidemic to a few groups, to a hub in which people coming to Quest became community members forming a healing place of support. Lucas and I both volunteered at Quest every day. In addition, I would see patients who had insurance who could pay, as Quest needed money to function.

How AIDS Work Changed Me

Through participation at Quest, I personally felt called to live a more authentic life. With this realization, I found that my marriage of 25 years could not withstand the changes. I addressed the guidance I received in the shared dream with Lucas, in which I needed to have a more egalitarian role. My initial marriage contract was like that of my parents, where my mother was disempowered. She was careful not to have too many needs or a voice. I knew I could not live my life following this example and still be true to myself. Still, it was not an easy decision. If I divorced, Quest would lose the funding my marriage had provided. I did not need to earn a living, as my husband provided the money for us to live on, and he paid the rent for our space. As Lucas and I committed to getting together every day to do meditation and ask for guidance for creating a healing center, I experienced being seen, appreciated, and loved in a way that I had never known. I continued to feel burdened at home by Leo's needs and his irritability and rage. The contrast of sharing from the heart with innocence, vulnerability, and openness that I experienced with Lucas, Jack, Tom, and others was obvious.

Around this time, I had the privilege of watching a transformation in Bud, a nurse who had come to Quest and worked in a hospital until he could no longer do his job. Bud was a man who had many symptoms from his advancing illness. In a psychodrama, it became clear to Bud that he was not in love with his partner of 13 years, and that he stayed in the relationship because he wanted to be sure he had someone who would care for him as he died. With support from his community, he left that relationship. Bud's willingness to let go of what felt deadening and to live fully with whatever time he had inspired me, helping me to be able to leave a marriage where the changes I was making were very threatening to my husband. I knew I could not go back to a comfortable middle-class life. I was an activist and would be involved in ways that my marriage could not withstand. I wanted relationships where it was safe to be vulnerable, to have needs, and to dream, and I wanted to live my life fully.

Shortly thereafter, I had another powerful community experience that brought clarity to me. I was with Brandt, who was dying of cryptococcal meningitis and had slipped into a coma. His partner Guy created a beautiful room for Brandt, and asked that we, his friends, take turns holding space for Brandt. He arranged for those who had the strength and willingness in our community to sit in pairs with Brandt for four-hour shifts. Guy asked that we come early, to enter into a meditative state before entering Brandt's space. When Lucas and I took our turn, I felt incredibly moved with love for Brandt, for Guy, for Lucas, and for all things. When Brandt's parents arrived, Guy asked them to take time to get to a quiet state in preparation for seeing their son. I was deeply moved by the role that Guy had as guardian for his beloved Brandt, and the peaceful, loving atmosphere he created for Brandt's death. I began to formulate more clearly how I wanted to die. I knew that if I were to die and Leo and I were still married, I had to have a plan for keeping him out of the room so I could die staying with my own experience. I knew that my husband, as a medical doctor, might force me to have heroic measures or treatments I might not want. I also knew, as I thought about my own death, that I had to leave my marriage. I wanted to be loved and valued and to die with a field of loving support for my safe passage and for me.

The decision to follow my inner guidance, even when it meant I would jeopardize the material comforts and mainstream validation, was hard, but I am so glad that my community of people with AIDS modeled for me a courageous way of living and dying. I saw that when those in our Quest community realized they might have less than two years to live, they often made big changes that would deepen their relationships, though these decisions often threatened their material comfort. I am grateful that I ultimately did the same.

Several men in the Quest community bought me Tina Turner shoes and music. They let me know that living fully was an important value for all of us, and that included me. Staying in a marriage that needed to end because of money was against our principles. Trust in following inner guidance, and the willingness to address obstacles while looking for solutions, was part of our foundation. I divorced and we did not have money for rent for Quest. I lived in a basement and worked as a psychotherapist to be able to provide needed funds for our mission. It was a difficult decision, but I realized that with a few silk and velvet fabrics, even my basement dwelling could become a comfortable place.

Lucas had been with me, cared for me, through many deaths. We would be present together through a beloved community member's death. I would be holding space for the dying person, breathing with them and creating a quiet zone of safety and love. After the person's death and our closure with those present, Lucas would take me to a cozy restaurant on 23rd Avenue, near Forest Park. Often I would not have had a meal for quite a while as I focused on the needs of the person dying. After we ate, Lucas and I would walk in the woods on a trail in the park that led to a bench near a stream. We would sit together on that bench until I could come back to myself, to my grief and pain over the loss of someone I deeply cared about and the tragedy of AIDS. Finally, I could cry, and Lucas and I comforted each other. I experienced such wonderful kindness and loving support that sustained me and restored me for the next deaths that would happen. I never let myself look at the likelihood that Lucas would die, and I could not imagine the Quest community or my work without him.

I spent more and more time working with our community, and my private practice where I was making money became less and less. With our 501(c)3 status we could apply for grants and government funding. Our main focus remained on exploring healing, putting into practice what seemed useful, and sharing information with each other. We learned about a nonprofit organization called AIDS, Medicine, and Miracles that had yearly gatherings where many healers spoke and powerful forms of healing were presented. We submitted a proposal to present our guided imagery work, and it was accepted. Lucas and I presented at AIDS, Medicine, and Miracles, where we were inspired by Gabriel Roth's ecstatic dance work, sweat lodges, and chanting, and brought those experiences back to Quest. By that time, we had shifted into being a wellness center with integrative healthcare and with community as an essential ingredient.

The Project Quest Community Takes Flight

As Quest unfolded, the work was filled with challenges, but many people felt moved to participate. We were open to the ideas and thoughts of our participants and a process of co-creation. It was clear from working with people with AIDS that they often felt disempowered by the medical system and not included as partners in understanding and making decisions. Learning to connect, to listen within, and to trust inner wisdom and guidance was a lost art and skill that needed to be revived. Living with inner guidance and the power of community spirit was an essential part of Quest.

Graham, a psychotherapist in his twenties living with AIDS, came in the early 1990s as a recent graduate of a therapy training program. Graham was as passionate about providing therapy that touched the inner experience of our community members as I was. He brought knowledge about funding and infrastructure that Quest was lacking, along with willingness, generosity of spirit, and a good sense of humor. We were known in the AIDS community as an alternative way to get help, rather than just depending on doctors and hospitals. Graham had his own challenges, and the intensity of the work took courage. He was very involved as members of our community would become very sick and die. Having a therapist who was living with AIDS brought profound understanding that our folks experienced as amazing and beneficial.

In the early 1990s, Graham joined Robin and me at psychodrama retreats. Most retreats would have 12 to 15 people plus facilitators. We would stay in a house that was donated for use by friends or people who had heard of our work and wanted to help. Each of us took on tasks such as determining together where people would sleep, the schedule we would keep, and cooking and cleanup. Issues and conflicts would arise, and we would address them, developing the skills for honest communication.

Robin, Graham, and I planned a special long-term experience we called "Changing Patterns/Changing Lives." It started with a retreat that took place on Orcas Island. We knew that the journey itself was part of the healing. Twenty-eight of us attended this unforgettable journey, caravanning to the ferry.

Bonnie Blackwolf, a woman from the Blackfeet tribe, was in vulnerable health with Hep C and HIV. She was a spokeswoman nationwide for women with HIV and part of our clan. She had been a trumpet player in New York City when she contracted AIDS, returning to the West Coast as her illness progressed. Bonnie did not join us for our group gathering the first morning after our arrival. When I checked on her, I found her still in bed. As I tried to rouse her, I realized she was in a coma and I could see blood. Robin and Graham came to her room, and we decided I should take her to the ferry and to a hospital in Anacortes. We informed all those present of our plan and the need to be present with love and support for Bonnie. In moments, the community mobilized. Jessie played his flute, and Bonnie was carried out by those who could help in a spontaneous ceremony. Graham and Robin stayed with the community while I drove with Debbie, Bonnie's dear friend. Debbie sat beside Bonnie, softly talking and singing. We arrived at the hospital, and Bonnie was initially in the ICU. Meanwhile, Graham and Robin led the retreat, and the experience with Bonnie inspired deep and meaningful work. This event triggered fear in each person with AIDS, in facing the stark reality of sickness, helplessness, and the specter of death.

It turned out that Bonnie had gone into a coma with the advent of her period. With HIV and Hep C, her body could not stand the extra burden. She came out of the hospital at the same time our community was heading home from the retreat and shared with us a vision of the work she needed to do before she died—which included getting her band members from New York City together for closure they never had, and for one last concert. This happened and was healing for all who were involved. Bonnie also saw herself in the white beaded buckskin dress she would wear at her death. She died on December 1, World AIDS Day, in her buckskin dress, surrounded by music, prayer, and love. Our community once again supported the special journey of each individual, and the wisdom and love that vulnerable sharing and witnessing engenders.

A Deep Loss

At Quest, the work was filled with challenges. Receiving the information about testing HIV positive was terrifying, so our community included people who were newly traumatized by their diagnosis and those who were sick and dying as our members. Those with AIDS would face health crises, and we would organize around how to get people to appointments, care for those who became incapacitated, and cook for those in need, as well as generally give support. Many people felt moved to participate and volunteered as professionals with skills such as music therapy, massage, Reiki, or doing office work. We were open to the ideas and thoughts of our participants and a process of co-creation.

We provided support for each person to address habits and patterns that limited health. This was achieved by emphasizing healthy eating, the value of exercise, and of living an authentic, engaged life. Even with all that we were doing, over 40 of our community members died. We stayed connected with love and support through people's illnesses and dying processes. The early days at Quest were often filled with heartache and heartbreak, but also with the strength that love brings. Quest provided a deeply grounded experiential understanding of life and death. We fully embraced the awareness that in knowing death, we live our lives more fully.

Lucas had experienced various opportunistic infections, and his spirit and the love from his community pulled him through. But in October 1995 Lucas was wasting and his health was failing. We had a gathering with over 70 people present. Each person was able to tell Lucas how his life had impacted theirs. As Lucas grew sicker, he had times of becoming very frustrated, scared, and angry. He had lost his handsome, boyish look and was emaciated with sunken features, familiar changes we had witnessed with community members moving into "the cascade of events" as systems stop working and death becomes more imminent.

I loved Lucas, and I too felt scared as he grew weaker. Somehow, I think that we both believed there would be a miracle and he would live, but now we knew he was dying. In his dying process, he began to distance from me. He spent more and more time with Robin and her family. I knew he was loved, understood, and safe with Robin, but I missed him. When we were together, he would express his irritability and rage. I tried to accept it, knowing that anger is often present in the dying process. Sometimes Lucas would berate me over the privilege of my teenage children. I could listen and understand, but I was shutting down and so was he.

One day as we were out for a walk, he was especially angry. When we returned to the house where he was staying, he punched the window, shattering the glass, his hand, and shattering my heart. His life felt out of control and I felt myself pulling away from him. I so wanted to help him feel safe and supported, but my own history made me feel scared. His reaction to his rapidly failing health was so different than I had expected. Lucas had been with me, cared for me through so many deaths. I never let myself look at the likelihood that he would die, and I could not imagine Quest or my work without him.

Lucas died in March of 1996. Tragically, he was too sick to be able to handle the antiretroviral medications that had recently come out. He had experienced encephalitis before and hated the treatment that consisted of daily IVs. He referred to the IVs as "shake and bake," as he said the symptoms of chills and fever and feeling awful were more than he wanted to endure. I had been devastated that Lucas, my soulmate and friend, the one with whom I had shared my heart and my dreams in the deepest way, was dying. He had been leaving me over the last months of his life. I was deeply saddened and hurt. I somehow did not envision him dying. In my thoughts about him being sick, I imagined I would care for him. It was painful for me that he did not want me around him as he became weaker and sicker. As the person closest to him, I became the safest one for him to express his rage to, and I was not able to be present in the way that I wanted to be. I always loved him, and I knew he loved me, but neither of us had the capacity to stay accepting as his health failed.

Like so many deaths, Lucas's was painful and unforgettable. He woke from a coma one day and demanded to play chess. He could hear private conversations in other parts of Robin's house and demanded to be included in everything that was happening around him even though he was in terrible pain. Robin, Jack, Lucas's partner Michael, and his friend Lusana were with him throughout his dying time. I was at AIDS, Medicine, and Miracles, the inspiring retreat where Lucas and I had co-presented for the last three years. I felt his spirit and a deep grief at this loss. I would not have had the courage to embark on this journey and the healing it brought for each of us without the sincerity and spirit of this amazing man who had been a teacher and friend.

Caring for those who became too weak to care for themselves, supporting people through the dying process, and having memorials were all part of our culture. Having fun, joking, and humor were also part of our community. As more people were living with the advent of antiretroviral medication, we courageously rented a beautiful facility with hot springs called Breitenbush and organized four-day healing retreats that brought people with HIV from all over the state to experience psychodrama, Native American sweat lodges, ecstatic dance, and community. A number of people from rural areas had never been able to be open about their illness and felt the healing and relief of sharing and learning together. These retreats, which we did for seven years, would have 150 people, with many practitioners who paid to come to provide treatments for free to those who were ill. The joy, laughter, and level of sharing would never be forgotten. I loved these gatherings and missed Lucas. I knew how much he would have loved these four-day events, which culminated in a talent show with a drag queen hostess and many surprises.

Community Ethos

Mutuality became a grounding principle in having our community be healthy. A formal therapist role frequently does not hold that concept. The therapist is defined as the empowered one who can provide needed guidance and support for the client. When we, in therapeutic roles, are honest and vulnerable appropriately, trust can deepen and those seeking help can be empowered. Mutuality involves bringing your full person present for yourself and for the relationship. The intersubjectivity of our relationships is an approach to healing that is as important in the here and now as it was in the early days of AIDS. It requires deepening to understand humanity as the human family that you are a part of, living as an authentic person. The construct holds how to live from "who I am" rather than "what I am," and to engage as a community that holds this value.

When I live from "who I am," I am vulnerable in a much greater way than from the construct that comes from "what I am," which holds a more clearly defined role. We used the experience that we shared with the AIDS crisis as a wake-up call to vulnerability, truthfulness, and love. The AIDS crisis/Quest experience holds a model of vulnerable people in a crisis committing more deeply to showing up. Instead of jumping to "every man for himself," we brought out at Quest that "we are in it together." It asked that each of us face the obstacles that come when you make that commitment. If a member of our community was dying, my inner guidance let me know that it was important that I stay engaged with the process, which might take days. Other responsibilities would need to wait. We faced judgments and sometimes ridicule from others as we veered from the mainstream, but it didn't sway our resolve. Some doctors considered acupuncture, guided imagery, and even eating a healthy diet as a waste of time. Living so closely with love and heartfelt connection to beloved people, men and women, with the reality of AIDS and death changes one's perceptions.

Often we develop automatic ways of processing, acting, and reacting that we are taught by society and other paradigms of power from a young age. Listening from within requires stepping out of automatic reactions and living in the moment. Quest developed a model of stepping back and getting perspective. Those who stayed asked questions that spurred critical thinking such as:

"Who am I and who is my community?"
"Does my doctor include me as a partner in developing my treatment?"
"Is the way I am with myself, my family, and my work life authentic?"

This book describes a model of people, initially those living with HIV, but later expanded to other life-challenging and chronic illnesses, and finally to all who seek "wellness-based" healthcare and community. Through this model, we developed personal resilience alongside community strength and spirit. Looking at long-term survival, we explored what it means and the barriers that exist. We learned to really see and be willing to step forth and say, "The emperor has no clothes." It became apparent that there are so many ways of acting and reacting. The "emperor" here refers to a way of showing up that lacks critical thinking and authenticity.

I learned in my early life to be guarded and careful. In entering a new experience, I scanned to see how I was supposed to look and act. I would guess what parts of me needed to be kept out of sight, and what parts would be acceptable.

This skill, learned in my family and conservative community growing up, became automatic. The injunction for life became: Do not be yourself, be what the "rules" require. If you veer too much from the social norm, you will become an outsider. Accept the rules and act accordingly.

Living Life Fully with AIDS

Living life fully was definitely part of the mission statement of Quest. After experiencing ecstatic dance with Gabriel Roth at AIDS, Medicine, and Miracles and feeling the aliveness that came from it, we Questers began to dance. We experienced the power of a sweat lodge with Two Foxes, and many of our community would choose to attend and find this spiritual practice brought clarity, guidance, and healing. Different traditions and modalities helped us tap into experiences of knowing: being more in touch with what felt true and listening to our soul clarity. Living life with spirit has always been a core Quest value. We found that mask making, art, music, poetry, and the creative process brought more life. Our psychodrama retreats continued to have an important place. We explored early traumas in sacred space, fear in the here and now, and how to be true to ourselves, both in solitude and in relationships.

As the antiretroviral medications were coming out in 1995, many people had been on a course that would end in death. When they began to take the new medications, many had to make a U-turn back to a different focus, that of living. In our Quest community, Ken Ballard had prepared for his death by getting a large-screen TV to watch the World Series. He had always loved baseball. Much to his surprise, with the advent of the medications, he began to feel better and his T-cell count went up. He realized he was going to live. In this realization, he decided to form Team Quest, a softball team. More people stopped smoking, started exercising, and eating better from softball than from my therapy sessions! Team Quest was a hit. It had gay men and heterosexual men and women with HIV all playing softball in the Gay City League with Ken as their coach. They lost their first 30 games, but all had fun, and Ken won a prize for coach of the year. There was amazing healing in playing softball!

Over and over, we listened to what our community said they needed, and co-created Quest. It was a program that valued the greater wisdom that came from shared and sacred space. Richard Francis led us in poetry and writing, and would have folks make sugar skulls and celebrate our friends and family who died at a yearly Day of the Dead ceremony. He also developed and edited our quarterly newsletter. We had music, including a didgeridoo player and singing bowls. We would lie on the floor and feel our very cells come alive as we immersed ourselves in the sounds and felt the healing energy of these collective experiences.

Greg Fowler had been near death on numerous occasions, even after the antiretrovirals came out. He realized he needed a goal to get his strength back.

He followed up on the Team Quest concept by proposing that we climb Mount Rainier. This would require a lot of endurance, strength building, and exercise. He was able to enlist the help of a local gym, where at no cost we had weekly workouts together. I was part of the Team Quest Mountain Climbing Crew. Of the 20 people from our group and 10 others who were in the party of 30 who made the climb with trained mountaineers, only two people actually reached the summit, both of whom had AIDS.

Overall, it became clear that each person has a "Wise Self" or "Inner Healer" who can be cultivated and provide guidance for living more fully as one's "True Self." We have all learned to disconnect and to check out, to listen to the voices of the so-called authorities about what we should and should not do. In moving away from this, we found a way of living, an essence or spirit within each of us that grew more into the foreground and became a stronger guiding, compassionate force in our lives. When we come together as a community and listen together for guidance, we know much more about how to resolve issues and conflicts and we develop a sense of greater trust, safety, and belonging. We are here for ourselves and for each other. Our decisions and choices need to keep both things in mind.

Death

Sogyal Rinpoche's *The Tibetan Book of Living and Dying* came out in 1993. I read it and reread it several times, as it offered guidelines for being with dying people that made dying a part of life. Death is an experience each of us will face that so often is put far out of awareness. It was always a powerful presence at Quest. We learn in Western culture to defend against it—as if that will keep it from happening. This book spoke to the value of bringing the awareness of death for each of us into the foreground. Lucas and I attended a ten-day retreat where these principles were taught. At our own retreats we would have a sacred space dedicated to dying and those who had died, and a sacred space dedicated to living fully. The awareness of death brought a different relationship with time, and the value of resolving relationship issues and defining more clearly one's dreams. People at Quest cared for one another. We helped each other face barriers and move towards articulating and, when possible, realizing unlived dreams.

The spirit of authenticity, returning to the memory of wholeness, emerged for me as I struggled to show up in an uncharted territory and time, where terrible wasting illness and death were happening to a marginalized portion of our population. Death is a very powerful force, and in our early days the shadow of death was always present. We did not know who death would take next—which is a catalyst to finding one's inner truth. I was called to be present as persons of our community became really sick and were dying. Ben was a man in his late twenties who had been wasting and getting weaker. His health had been failing during the last two years. His community at Quest helped him role play, exploring his feelings and how to address his mother in his alienated family, and then other family members. We were all deeply moved when he actually talked with his mother and she wept. She came back into his life, as did other family members. When he slipped into a coma, his family came to be with him. I stayed present, not knowing that Ben's dying would take days.

We supported each other through this time. I shared the images he had been working with and his explorations of how he wanted things to be as he died. They shared the stories of his life, stories of him as the sweet child he had been. We created a field of love and support around him. Ben's death was very painful, but the effort he put forth to live as fully as he could every day taught me a lot. Being able to reconcile with his family was incredibly meaningful and so important to him and each of them, as we lived together through his death. I had no idea that his dying process would take so long, and that I would be spending three days and two nights in the apartment of a "client." I knew that I had made a promise to Ben to have his back and that I was required spiritually for Ben and for myself to stay present through the long and arduous process of his death. I felt a profound loss, but more a part of things than I ever had.

We often talked about dying at Quest, as we focused on living fully and developing the habits and traits of long-term survival. Exploring death and one's beliefs around it is one of those traits. Facing one's fear with curiosity, kindness, and awareness actually helps one live longer and with less anxiety.

There were many situations in dealing with dying people that had me face the reality of my own life and the lack of genuine understanding in how my husband and other family members and I had related to each other. My community had become the AIDS community, and I learned amazing lessons in courage and willingness to face enormous challenges: to not distract, check out, or run away.

Lucas's friend Bob was in the first group I led at Quest in the late 1980s. He had grown up in and out of foster care with a mother who'd been diagnosed with a serious mental illness, who often could not take care of her children. Bob used to bring in flowers to our sessions. He said that he helped out at a florist shop and could take pots of flowers and bouquets beyond their prime. Later, we learned that he took them from cemeteries, as he felt the living needed them more than the dead. When Bob moved in with a partner, he brought along his 20-pound cat and his grandmother, who was 90 years old. Bob died a very different death than Brian or Brandt. He had been living in Hawaii, and upon his return to Portland was immediately hospitalized. After being discharged from the hospital, within 12 hours he was running a high fever. He returned to the hospital, and I was notified that he was dying of septicemia. His ex-partner, Greg, who was Bob's true love, showed up at the same time I did. Bob was fully awake and aware. Meanwhile, his grandmother had a heart attack and was in the ER. Bob asked that I keep his mother out of his room, and I was pleased to be able to protect him in this way. I supported her in having a special room where members of

Bob's community who knew her were able to be with her, offering prayers that had her feel engaged and included. In Bob's hospital room we entered into a sacred space. Bob had developed a healing image of a heron landing on Lake Vancouver that helped him manage stress. Bob used that image and felt the love and support from those of us who were present. He never went into a coma, but suddenly the room became light, and he was gone. We stayed with him in prayer and song. I had come to know more fully the amazing variation in the ways people die and the feeling of grace and mystery that I felt in someone's passing from this life.

Quest Now

Quest has survived through time, more than 30 years. It is an integrative health center that is wellness focused and fosters the power of community. Every program has peer mentors on staff, as we learned how much trust there can be, and how effective, when those seeking services are served by people who share their story and therefore can provide understanding and support. The organization still has the goal of treating all people, especially those who are marginalized, with traditional, complementary, and alternative treatments, and providing support for dying peacefully and living fully. Through the process of creating Quest, the invitation and my willingness to enter into the world of people living with AIDS, my life was changed forever. I was not infected, but deeply affected at a cellular and a soul level.

It has been an enormous challenge to keep the wisdom of those early times alive and central to Quest in the here and now. The spirit of wonderful people, many who died, is a foundation that still exists and that we draw from. Quest was able to have David Eisen, who had been the executive director of a large drug and alcohol treatment program that used acupuncture, become our executive director. In 1992 when I got divorced, he provided housing for Quest in the basement of his program in downtown Portland. He helped us survive some really hard times. We developed a trusting relationship in the early 1990s when he rented us space for $200 a month, with utilities included. He felt the Quest spirit and years later, in 2005, he decided to join us, as we needed leadership to create the infrastructure of a business.

Quest survived for years because it spoke to the people who were involved, and we faced our various challenges together. I lacked the skills to develop a structure and the relationships with funders that are necessary for a stable and thriving nonprofit organization. David understood the spirit of Quest, and also the desperate need for stability and funding. As a doctor of Chinese medicine and a passionate health practitioner, he brought a very different awareness to his role. He wanted a place where he could continue to be a practitioner and use his experience and wisdom to help Quest become a truly integrative clinic. He realized the importance for our folks with HIV and for people living with life-challenging illnesses and chronic conditions to have innovative programs with evaluations that would show results that funders needed—such as fewer trips to the ER, fewer symptoms, and more satisfaction among clients.

With David's leadership, we were able to develop a needed alcohol and drug treatment program with acupuncture, yoga, and naturopathic treatment, and really put our integrative approach into practice with results. We chose as our targeted communities the LGBTQ+ community, people living below the poverty level who rarely are able to receive powerful treatments that complement the medical model, and people from all walks of life who seek wellness-based healthcare—which is very different from a disease-based model. Quest continues to have a strong program for HIV services. We currently have the only psychosocial program for HIV-positive women in the state of Oregon. Our HIV program uses peer mentors and continues to rely on the input and collaboration of our community. Quest developed an alcohol and drug treatment program as well, because for many, addiction stood in the way of healing. While still in the nineties our board, which mainly consisted of persons with HIV, decided that we should be open to all who were seeking "wellness-based healthcare" with a focus on the LGBTQ+ community.

The approach of listening to each person, with an openness to be in community with others, cooking, exercising, grieving losses, and sharing from the heart continues. Quest psychodrama retreats bring early participants, now often dealing with aging, present with the Quest community that is ever developing and changing. We continue to find the strength that comes from bearing witness to human struggles and triumphs, and sensing the ever-present path with heart, available to all. We still find the "magic" in love and the invitation to each person to a healing path of deeper consciousness.

Quest has been recognized by government funding sources as an effective model of healthcare. This year we have been invited to support rural counties in providing services for LGBTQ+ folks using telehealth and on-site approaches. We organized various special services for vulnerable communities during the COVID-19 quarantine and continue building safe and supportive services for our trans community members. During the COVID-19 pandemic, a long-term survivor of HIV, Christian, who had been living with cancer, experienced heart failure. Rents in Oregon have greatly increased, and he could not pay the rent to continue living in his apartment. He reached out to Mira, a woman he knew from Quest retreats, and asked if he could stay in an apartment that she had been using as a storage space in her garage. She discussed it further with him and agreed. It took a number of different Quest community members to go through Christian's accumulated items and help him downsize so he could move. Others helped clear space and with Mira's help, Christian moved in. Mira told me that sharing her backyard with Christian helped both of them during the COVID-19 quarantine. Together they watched birds and learned the art of Bonsai. Christian elected to have a special surgery on his heart, hoping it would give him more time to work through his bucket list, but he died the week following his surgery. It was heartwarming to see that the spirit of Quest was vibrant and present as we celebrated Christian's life and felt the deep grief and loss with his death.

Our healthcare system today is in desperate need of a community approach with vital energy, innovative solutions, love, and compassion. The model of treating people in crisis and ignoring disenfranchised groups must be addressed, and the Quest way holds some fundamental guidelines. A more compassionate model that is less based on colonial top-down care, offering more mutuality, is needed. Listening within, rather than our cultural model of people in general being plugged into their phones and electronic devices, is key. Cultivating the willingness to be vulnerable and to take risks was very important during the AIDS crisis and continues to be essential. We hold a vision of inspiration for changing our broken healthcare system as it exists today.

Quest, with David's leadership and the help of our community allies, was able to purchase a building large enough for all of our programs to be under one roof, and it now has more than 75 employees. I had begun to build mutual aid groups, so that as we moved into a new space with a beautiful kitchen and large room for dining for our weekly community dinner, people would know each other and feel a sense of belonging. Our "Quest" to support each person and the "Common Unity" of the community still has a strong beating heart.

Chapter 5

Rethinking of Boundaries and Professionalism During a Crisis

Graham Harriman

I joined Quest as a contracted therapist in 1992. Quest had just moved to a space in the basement of a single-room occupancy hotel, sharing space with a substance use treatment program. Volunteers came together with donated plywood, doors, drywall, and carpet to create a sanctuary for people with AIDS. We made do with what little we had as an organization at the time. My office was the intake room. There were no windows, but colorful decorations, tasteful lighting, and a lending library of donated therapy books greeted newcomers.

Sexual Health and so-called "Addiction"

One of the first requests from the Quest community was to initiate services to address sexual health and sexual compulsion. This was due to the ongoing challenges of being HIV positive and how that was affecting their sexual relationships, their health, and persistent feelings of shame and guilt. As the gay, male, HIV-positive therapist, I would be most able to understand this dynamic, given my experience and understanding of sex and gay culture. I enrolled in a week-long training with Patrick Carnes to understand the theory and treatment of sex addiction/sexual compulsion. The model at the time was based on Carnes's book *Out of the Shadows* (Carnes, 1983). Treatment on psychopathology was focused on the premise that the symptoms of sexual compulsivity/sex addiction were aberrant behaviors that needed to be removed from a person's experience. The model recognized personal trauma, sexual, physical, and verbal abuse, as a leading factor for most who experience sexual compulsivity. A family history of substance abuse, overeating, gambling, and other compulsive behaviors was prevalent among persons with sexual compulsion, leading to learned behaviors to manage feelings such as anxiety and depression. The treatment of sex addiction therefore focused on finding sources of compulsive behaviors and identifying triggers to limit behaviors labeled as addictive.

This sex addiction model, however, attempts to limit sexual behaviors as a means of controlling compulsive behavior but in doing so it ignores cultural attitudes towards sex that inhibit free expression. Additionally, the United States'

DOI: 10.4324/9781003386339-8

mainstream culture retains strict limits on acceptable and unacceptable behaviors and controls individuals through shame and marginalization. Gay men with AIDS experience marginalization through sexism and heterosexism, stigma, and subsequently are relegated to the periphery of society. The sex lives of gay men are outside of the norm at its most fundamental level. This is in contrast to a culture founded on sexism that is at the root of heterosexism and transphobia. As people with HIV, we paid for heterosexism through cultural ostracism and staggering governmental silence, resulting in the death of hundreds of thousands of people in the 1980s and 1990s. Codified lists of acceptable and unacceptable sexual practices used in sex addiction treatment didn't fit well with the needs of gay men seeking sexual health. This rigidity had the risk of retraumatizing and shaming individuals through mirroring mainstream culture's discomfort with gay sex, including anal sex and non-monogamous relationships.

I experienced cultural ostracism myself as an HIV-positive gay man. I came out to my family in the late 1980s, as part of a many-year process of learning to be comfortable with myself and with my sexuality. I felt the ostracism of friends who disconnected from me in college after I came out. I learned to connect socially with friends who had similar experiences of marginalization due to heterosexism, racism, classism, sexism, and other mechanisms of social control.

After my first initial relationship with a man in college, I met a guy in a bar that I saw for several months. I remember being determined to make the relationship work, regardless of some clear signs that we lacked connection. I learned in the most difficult way that I didn't know how to set a boundary, and I didn't know how to stand up for myself. I know now that I should have left that relationship long before I did, but I wanted acceptance. Three and a half months into the relationship he raped me. I still remember not understanding what was happening in that moment. I do remember the pain I felt, and his lack of concern or interest in me, or that he was inflicting that pain. I remember knowing that I was most certainly HIV positive, testing HIV positive three months later. I think his act of raping me was a combination of a desire to inflict pain on someone close to him, discomfort with his AIDS diagnosis, and a deep desire to not deal with it alone. I did learn that he had shared his HIV status and his health challenges with others over a year before, information he never disclosed to me. I share this to clarify my own struggles with sexual health that included internalized AIDS phobia and homophobia, heterosexism, rape trauma, my desire for connection, uncertainty about how to ask for what I needed, and how to set limits for my own protection. After my diagnosis, it became a compounded challenge to know who accepted me for who I am, and who would see me as a vector for the disease. Four years later I trained in sex addiction and led the sex addiction group, with the knowledge of how I had managed, for better and worse, my own sexual health decision making.

I began leading the group four years after my HIV-positive diagnosis, after some time to process my experience, being further along in my training as a psychotherapist. At first, I tried to adhere to the model of sex addiction, but over time I understood the most salient issue for group members was the struggle for connection to an inner self—a deeper understanding of wants and yearnings, to address loneliness, shame, connection, and the pursuit of unconditional love. Group members sought to understand their internalized AIDS phobia and homophobia, and responses to trauma. Through work in the group and psychodrama retreats, acupuncture, and other holistic healing treatments, many participants came to know that they had been acting on their passion in altered states of trauma. These altered states were barriers to experiencing the sensuality and connection they yearned for. The group functioned best when participants shared their stories in their most raw form. This was contrary to the sex addiction model that neatly placed sexual practices in boxes of acceptability and unacceptability, boxes known all too well by gay men who internalized society's beliefs that their sex lives were amoral, dirty, and promiscuous. I began to learn through group member experiences that the work required a spiritual element—an honest connection to self that helped the group participants to understand their longings, passion, and their pursuit of life, with meaning, purpose, unconditional love, and connection.

It was within these early experiences as a group therapist that I realized the many dimensions of dual-relatedness that I engaged in as a gay man living with HIV in a small, affected community. One of the clearer examples of my management of dual roles is when I first met Joseph (his name is changed to maintain anonymity) when he came for his intake. In his intake I helped him get a sense of what he needed from Quest and how we could best help him. At the time, he had been living with HIV, and hepatitis C, for over ten years. He also had several years of not using methamphetamine, yet he continued to experience sexual health challenges, unsure of how to connect to other gay men without sex, while yearning for deepened, meaningful relationships with men. Post intake, Joseph joined the sex addiction group I was leading at the time. He was committed to the group and shared his experiences freely, knowing that it was important for his healing, and in doing so it supported the group's process.

After a period of time in the group, he also joined other efforts at Quest, including the Changing Patterns/Changing Lives group, which was formed to initiate long-term changes in social behaviors and improve health and well-being. At the time, my ex-partner also joined this group. Joseph and my ex-partner became close through the group work, and later married. I continued to be a co-therapist for their group. Being a therapist in the community with Joseph, and my ex-boyfriend/Joseph's husband, I adapted to a revision of boundaries in the small community. Joseph became a central community member—participating in groups, psychodrama retreats, managing the Team Quest baseball team, volunteering in the office, and later serving on the board.

My therapeutic relationship with Joseph is only one of *many* examples where traditional professional boundaries were impossible. The requirement that the therapist maintain a blank slate and have no outside relationship with the client was unrealistic amidst an accelerating AIDS crisis and within my subculture of gay men with AIDS in a small city. The time and place necessitated that we recreate therapeutic relationships as we went along. The work called for conscious reflection and an understanding of the goals of community-oriented therapy. I therefore sought support from my colleagues to ensure that I remained in a role of service to Joseph and other clients so that I could keep the community members' well-being in perspective. At Quest, we met as colleagues from a variety of orientations—psychotherapists, substance use counselors, nutritionists, and medical staff—to review cases and receive insight. It was in the crisis environment working in the midst of an epidemic that we learned how best to respond to the needs of our clients and community as they arose.

Reorienting Professional Boundaries

Much of the literature on the dangers of dual relationships is based on sexual dual relationships (Gabriel, 2005). Conservative values regarding sexual dual relationships led to a prohibition on all dual relationships. This ethical mandate does not recognize the kinds of mutuality and overlapping dual roles that often exist in a small community experiencing a crisis or catastrophe. This restricted understanding of therapist/client relationships inhibits the psychotherapist from being able to communicate intentional loving regard with clients in a landscape of death, dying, and living fully. Indeed, the traditional psychotherapeutic relationship between client and therapist has been mechanized and ignores essential therapeutic elements related to a client's mental health, relationship, positive regard, care, and mutuality.

Reorienting professional boundaries came with shame, disapproval, and some hostile responses from those who questioned anyone not adhering to traditional professional roles. Lynne Gabriel studied and published more on dual relationships, over a decade after our work at Quest, opening the door to constructive discourse regarding the need for reviewing overlap in boundaries that occur more often than many admit. She offers a few supportive guidelines for dual relationships such as recognition of dual relationships between therapist and client; reviewing practice and motives for dual relationships; use of supervision; and aiming to be a "good versus a malevolent influence" (Gabriel, 2005, p. 129). We had already intuitively discovered many of these supportive elements in our clinical practices that we are just now articulating. Our practices were conscious, intentional, always non-sexual, and guided by benevolent values. We were open, and not clouded by secrecy or hindered by shame.

Feminist psychology served as the theoretical basis of my work, in particular Jessica Benjamin's groundbreaking work on client/therapist mutuality (1988). I first came across her work in a philosophy class during my undergraduate degree. Her ability to develop a post-Freudian analysis of the importance of mutuality in relationships as a therapeutic tool stuck with me. Benjamin challenged the strict line between therapist as all-knowing practitioner (and object) and the client as the receiver of knowledge (subject). She viewed the relationship between therapist and client as a therapeutic tool, and a means of co-creativity. Her work was a necessary approach in an era where we all needed each other during the rapidly escalating AIDS crisis. Hierarchy and patriarchal assumptions were necessarily questioned as people with AIDS (PWA) faced their mortality.

My professional role as a therapist and my place in the community I lived in, and served, were inseparable. Indeed, I engaged in many dual relationships that included ex- partners, friends, friends of friends, and acquaintances of friends, most of whom shared my experience of being a person living with AIDS. Furthermore, I also participated in a number of Quest group climbing adventures, where we hiked and camped overnight, facing a challenge outside of ourselves as a metaphor for facing our challenge with the disease. Participating as a therapist living with AIDS helped model efficacy and mutual challenges/experiences with others in the community, and freed us from the diagnosis of AIDS and society's marginalization. The common experience of living with AIDS solidified supportive connections that endure to this day. At the same time, it proved to be a challenge developing therapeutic relationships.

My training as a psychotherapist did not prepare me for what was relationally needed during the AIDS crisis. I continued my own psychotherapy to raise my awareness about my physical, spiritual, and psychological challenges with AIDS, and to navigate the complexity of continual transferential and counter-transferential phenomena. With these dynamics, I established myself in the organization as a person living with AIDS, and as a psychotherapist, knowing that it required a unique relationship with the clients I served and a continued state of mindfulness of how I interacted with people with HIV (PWH) seeking my help. I sought support from colleagues daily to ensure I approached my work with clear intention and focus on the client, with a parallel focus on my own healing and health.

I struggled with my health for the first ten years of my living with AIDS, and my first eight years of being a therapist with people with HIV/AIDS. I came in and out of periods of wasting, where the body consumes its own stores of energy for survival, and developed multiple drug resistances. This was a common issue with those diagnosed early who developed resistance to classes of medications, as they were put on the market before effective combination therapies were developed. Additionally, I had poor liver and kidney function, which gave me severe fatigue, as a result of the earlier more toxic medications. I had persistent diarrhea due to poor immune function, and I was diagnosed with cytomegalovirus (CMV) in my eyes, which threatened my eyesight and required IV drips twice a day for 18 months. I continued to work during these challenges. I recall an AIDS retreat I co-led with Robin on Whidbey Island. The IV device was strapped to my body throughout the four days. My challenges living with AIDS were ever present in my role as a therapist and community member. In spite of my ongoing discomfort, Robin and I offered our comfortable bedroom to a couple who, when they arrived, discovered all of the full or queen-sized beds had already been taken. After much group processing, nobody wanted to give up their bed. The couple were cantankerous and worn down by disease, making it difficult for many to feel compassion for their need to sleep together as a couple. Robin and I couch surfed during the entire retreat, modeling a tenet of mutual aid that had not yet taken hold in the group.

I developed coping skills by being a part of a community through a combination of service and engagement with my fellow PWA. We shared information on treatments, alternative medicines, approved Western medicines, and clinical trials. I relied on my partner, my family, and close friends for support. In community, I learned to cook in a way that allowed me to gain the most healing from food and I surrounded myself with people who were seeking hope and stiving to survive.

I maintained a number of long-term friendships with PWA who managed their health challenges when treatment was scarce, and with them we continue to manage the current era of facing common comorbidities related to aging that have an earlier onset with PWH/A (Collins & Armstrong, 2020). An example is my long-term friendship with Gary (his name changed here for anonymity). Gary is another long-term survivor who has lived for years advocating for his treatment, partnering with his medical provider to make the most informed decisions to maintain his quality of life in the face of adversity. In the early years, we were both at Quest, and I was a therapist and PWA, and Gary was a PWA, client, and a community leader. We shared resources, lived experiences, and our successes and challenges of living with AIDS as we were both continually exploring limited treatment options. I learned how to advocate for myself because of his own tenacity and determination in seeking health and life. Gary was also the leader of many mountain expeditions with Team Quest, always seeking and never giving in to the challenges that AIDS presented; I thank him for modeling such determination. Oftentimes, we have reflected about how, in the early years, we had no idea we would live this long but our mutual support and knowledge of each other's stories throughout our lives with HIV/AIDS has helped us persist through our health challenges.

My relationship to the organization was different than that of others. I was a therapist, a gay white man, and I was living with AIDS. These identities were a part of my work and central to how I engaged with PWH. I was privileged because of my education, my income, and my race that allowed me more access to resources. Fortunately, I had emotional support from my partner at the time, Carlos. He was my foundation throughout the more difficult years and held an unfaltering belief in my future which I am thankful for to this day. My parents and siblings gave me unconditional love and helped me financially when I couldn't work enough to pay my living expenses. My graduate school education gave me an understanding of psychological research on hope and wellness that greatly benefited my search for stable health. I was challenged by my awareness of privilege in a society where resources were unequally available. Thus, I strove to be open to other's experiences and to recognize the similarities and differences from my own. Living with the disease was our common denominator.

I supported clients in their engagement with their medical providers, their challenges with income, work, and family support. I explored their life stories in a variety of settings, including psychodrama retreats and groups. Through psychodrama, we found new narratives of resilience and hope for sustaining life whenever possible. We lifted common experiences of group participants to foster empathy, group cohesion, and understanding. I recall Darryl, who had been living with AIDS for a decade when he first joined the Quest community. He came from a childhood of poverty and carried that with him through his adulthood, living on a limited income. In the first year of coming to Quest, he quickly saw the need for help in the office, and he began answering the phones, scheduling appointments, responding to emails, and managing donations and fundraisers. Darryl and I had a collegial office relationship, but he also participated in groups and psychodrama retreats. I specifically recall a psychodrama in which he described his lack of connection and lack of expectations for support. As he shared his inner world, group members had an opportunity to share their appreciation for his kindness, generosity, and dedication to the community. In that moment, for the first time, the veil of his loneliness was lifted. He recognized his connection to others. As he finished his psychodrama, I too had an opportunity to state my appreciation for his integrity, friendship as a colleague, and dedicated service to all of us in the community. I'll never forget that moment.

While I came from a place of strength, I too was weakened by the disease. From the beginning I knew that I needed to let down my guard and consciously think of what was therapeutic in terms of the boundaries I maintained. My vulnerability was a strength. All of those who came to see me for psychotherapy knew I was a person living with AIDS. When they saw me, in the 1990s, if they didn't know beforehand, they could have figured it out because of my appearance. I was gaunt, underweight, and for several years I was on IV medication for my CMV, as described above. Most clients sought me out as a therapist because I was living with HIV and doing this work. They saw me as one of their own, knowing that I could understand their experience in a way that others could not. My perspective came from *lived experience* of HIV, including its many health challenges, and this is what many sought. PWH who came to see me for therapy had a desire to live and to live fully.

My colleagues Lusijah and Robin had decades more experience as therapists than I did. I finished graduate school just a year before joining Quest. Nevertheless, the three of us approached the work as equals. They respected my newly acquired academic knowledge and experience with the disease, as a gay man *in* the community. I brought a unique and critical clinical perspective to the organization. We made decisions on how to co-facilitate groups and where to focus our energy when so much was competing for our attention. We shared information on what programs and approaches would be most useful for Quest in collaboration with community members. Our work demanded that we pull ourselves outside of the typical hierarchical structures of client/therapist relationships to respond to what was needed. We conveyed compassion and care in a world that had otherwise turned its head away from PWA. We strove to be an organization that could embrace community needs while engaging with traditional funding streams including federal Ryan White Part A, Medicaid, and private medical insurance.

We developed a model of care that was *radically client-centered* but also utilized these traditional revenue streams to support our psychotherapeutic work. We held community meetings to develop responsive programs that met the current life challenges and needs of all who participated. Quest intentionally focused on flexing traditional boundaries so that "clients" became participants and were encouraged to take positions of leadership of activities (team quest, mountain hiking, nutrition night, for instance), organizing fundraisers and our annual five-day retreat, *Living Fully*, at Breitenbush Hot Springs. We established ourselves as a unique organization based on integrity, radical client-centered work, and a beacon of hope for PWH and others with life-challenging illnesses. Our community members wanted to belong to come out of isolation as they had been alienated by society at large.

Spirit of the Times

Quest's reformulated therapeutic boundaries emerged in response to empowerment of disenfranchised community members in the age of AIDS. It was an era when power dynamics were questioned and bureaucracies were challenged amidst an epidemic that affected marginalized people and offered few, if any, effective treatments. The community grieved from multiple losses, isolation, shame, loneliness, and fear; there was hopelessness and instilled anger. These conditions fueled our advocacy for our rights as human beings. We were marginalized by a misinformed and uncaring society and entrenched apathy of local, state, and federal governments that only under pressure would pay for care for people who were gay, injection drug users, Black, Latino, and/or poor.

Quest developed its unique approach as a part of the zeitgeist of AIDS activism that arose in the 1980s and 1990s. Schulman elaborates on this point in her book *Let the Record Show*:

> … great leaps happen every 40 years or so. Unfortunately, they cannot be forced; they depend on the zeitgeist. … When the zeitgeist moment hits – and AIDS activism was one of those moments – there is a mass surge forward …
> (Schulman, 2020, p. xviii)

The HIV advocacy movement from its inception focused on the importance of the *empowerment of people with HIV* supporting each other in treatment decisions, in advocating for improvements in the FDA approval process, and in challenging the top-down doctor/patient paradigm. Seeking health was born from a desire to survive in a culture which left us on the margins to fight for ourselves. And fight for ourselves we did.

Without a viable treatment and federal support for treatment and care, the Denver Principles were created in 1983 to develop a narrative in opposition to mainstream society's treatment of PWA. The list of principles included recommendations for PWA which included: Be involved at every level of decision making: Serve on the boards of directors of provider organizations; Be included in all AIDS forums with equal credibility as other participants, to share your own experiences and knowledge" (Denver Principles, 1983). PWA were organizing a culture of mutual support and advocacy in the face of being cut out of any effort for assistance. All of us were frustrated and fighting for our lives and Schulman recognized that without "energy, currency, connection, assertion, insistence, and culturally recognizable imagination in coalition with those with less power, AIDS would have never been transformed" (2021, p. 24).

Our outrage creatively mobilized us in many ways. We challenged the roles and boundaries between those traditionally considered knowledgeable (medical doctors and the medical establishment) and those considered without knowledge (patient/client). In an era of limited treatment, Western medicine had almost nothing to offer PWA. For instance, AZT was the only antiretroviral in the early years, which was hastily approved based on one study that inaccurately showed differences in mortality between those receiving treatment and a placebo (Spins Staff, 2015). The headaches, muscle aches, and anemia side effects of the drug were intolerable. Peer networks across the United States were essential for our survival. We shared information about treatments and access to experimental treatments in newsletters created by such organizations as Project Inform and Treatment Action Group and buyers' clubs such as the Dallas Buyers' Club. These groups provided hope lifelines and allowed rapid sharing of life-saving information among PWH.

As a result of these efforts, the reorientation of the doctor/patient relationship in the early era of AIDS had a ripple effect throughout the medical system, including the related fields of nursing, social work, and psychotherapy. No longer could a provider rest on their authority as the holder of wisdom, knowledge, and healing. Without effective treatment, each of us was responsible for instilling hope and supporting our survival. Empowering ourselves through these grassroots movements reoriented our boundaries and became essential to our continued existence. From this perspective, we can better understand how the Quest community was a subversive community of care amidst a broader environment of carelessness. It was a radical shift from the assumptions and confines of commonly accepted therapeutic relationships.

Closing Thoughts

I worked consciously in my role as a gay man living with AIDS who was also a therapist in a community that sustained me. It became a continual challenge to understand the needs of the clients versus my disease process. I worked hard to be sure what I shared was for the client's therapeutic benefit as each of us faced the challenges of HIV. Each person was experiencing much of what I was experiencing, and our similarities filtered through their life stories and their dreams of having a more stable health and life situation. Their work with me facilitated their ability to make healthcare decisions, maintain relationships with their partners, friends, and family/chosen family, and manage self-care. Issues of abuse, betrayal, trauma, and substance use were intersectional complexities that had to be accounted for when managing the disease and often became a significant focus of the work. Most clients faced serious challenges to their health as they encountered opportunistic infections, treatment failures, and serious side effects from the earlier antiretrovirals. These side effects included anemia, uncontrolled diarrhea, kidney stones, fat loss and fat redistribution, and liver and kidney failure. When clients were hospitalized, or admitted to a hospice, our work continued. We didn't limit ourselves to office space or office hours. A collaborative supportive community cannot work only 9 to 5. We were all creatively engaged in the work as the crises escalated. When community members were sick, we worked together—therapists, colleagues, and peers—to deliver food, check in, advocate with medical providers, and conduct home and hospital visits.

At Quest, we learned how to work in community by the seat of our pants. *The crisis demanded that we not conduct business as usual.* Quest's unique culture insisted on being present as a professional and present as a human being. As a therapist, I wasn't expected to work eight hours with a break for lunch, seeing clients for a 50-minute hour. We responded to community needs as they arose, whether it was three-day weekend retreats or 90-minute sessions. Our working ethos was one where relationship and social support was an essential part of the psychotherapeutic process and we employed it in praxis. This required that we continually challenged the commonly upheld assumption that any dual relationship was a risk to clients and considered taboo in the psychotherapeutic profession. I worked to maintain therapeutic relationships with participants at Quest in several ways. I only conducted individual sessions with people with whom I had no other relationship with outside of therapy. Group work and retreat work tended to be the environments where traditional boundaries were most altered. People who served on the board, worked in the office, and were connected to me through friendship participated in retreats. Robin, Lusijah, and I negotiated these relationships with care as we thought through what was most beneficial to participants.

Relating to each other as human beings was essential to our healing. Relationship, support, sharing knowledge, experience, and connection were of utmost importance in this era of acute crises. We sought to look into the eyes of the other, to listen to pain and understand human suffering. A culture of care required that we create spaces (community meetings, groups, retreats) for all to voice their experience. The environment encouraged individuals to suggest projects/work/initiatives that would be beneficial as we collaboratively built a tiny empowering society. We met weekly to cook and share healthy congregate meals. We developed support groups which met without therapists to create systems of social support. We encouraged participants to freely give their time, skills, and resources to sustain the organization. Lusijah, Robin, and I had roles as therapists, but also contributed to the organization with our financial resources, time, and administrative support, among the many others who also helped maintain the organization.

As I look back and reflect 30 years later, I realize that we created a unique environment through the combination of people who came to Quest. There was an array of life experiences of gay men, women and heterosexual men who were living with AIDS that joined through a shared hope of living fully, surviving, dying well, and supporting each other through the physical challenges of AIDS. There were also many kinds of therapeutic agents who participated with skills in Eriksonian hypnotherapy, psychodrama, feminist psychology, alternative therapies such as acupuncture, massage, naturopathy, and nutrition, and who supported a healing environment specific to the needs of group in a time and a place. We have much to learn from what we learned then about caring as a community. We also have much to build on from what we developed.

References

Benjamin, J. (1988). *The Bonds of Love: Psychoanalysis, Feminism, and the Problem of Domination*. New York: Pantheon Books.

Carnes, P. (1983). *Out of the Shadows*. Minneapolis, MN: ComCare.

Collins, L. F. and Armstrong, W. S. (2020). What It Means to Age with HIV Infection: Years Gained Are Not Comorbidity Free. *JAMA Network Open*, 3(6), e208023. https://doi.org/10.1001/jamanetworkopen.2020.8023

Denver Principles (1983). https://actupny.org/documents/Denver.html. Accessed February 17, 2024.

Gabriel, L. (2005). *Speaking the Unspeakable: The Ethics of Dual Relationships in Counselling and Psychotherapy*. London and New York: Routledge.

Schulman, S. (2021). *Let the Record Show: A Political History of ACT UP New York, 1987–1993*. New York: Farrar, Straus and Giroux.

Spin Staff (2015). AIDS and the AZT Scandal: SPIN's 1989 Feature, 'Sins of Omission.' www.spin.com/2015/10/aids-and-the-azt-scandal-spin-1989-feature-sins-of-omission/. Accessed October 30, 2023.

Chapter 6

Group Psychotherapy, Psychodrama, and Community Building

Robin McCoy Brooks

Setting the Scene

Imagine a room filled with individuals who may not live through the winter. Imagine bearing all kinds of physical discomfort and shame for what is happening to your body, as well as uncertainty about your future except for impending death. Imagine the isolation of having a diagnosis in a broader society that negates the reality of AIDS. Imagine the terror and horror of watching your friends and lovers die before you. Imagine the experience of losing a way of life that is no longer available to you, as your identity group is being wiped out, and that society at large appears to not notice or care about. One sociodrama I led, for example, revealed that many of the attending 28 participants had lost from 10 to over 100 loved ones to AIDS. I describe this sociodrama in Chapter 3.

I recall the initial visceral reaction to my first experience of co-leading an HIV retreat. During the first session, I began to notice how my body was becoming increasingly bloated, as if I could explode from every orifice. During our first break, I quickly ran to the bathroom and vomited into the sink. My body was shaking. I was overcome by the incomprehensible effects of the disease on so many beautiful minds and bodies, all gathered in a single room. I was also humiliated and ashamed for not knowing what was happening in my own neighborhood. Hubris regulated my grandiosity. I was literally engulfed by a psychical emptying out. The Lacanian psychoanalyst Julia Kristeva refers to such moments as the "alterity of madness" or the "ground zero of psyche … spasms and vomit, repulsion, the retching that thrusts me to the side and turns me away from defilement, sewage and muck, a void improper and unclean" (Kristeva, 1987, p. 160). I wanted to run away from the evidence of my insularity, and I could not look away. I was powerfully moved by the immediacy of tenderness, a deep desire to live fully, the wicked humor and transparency that violently opened my heart, pulling me backwards into the hedges of AIDS. As I washed the vomit off my face, I looked into the mirror and privately asked myself, "Can I really do this?" Fierce tensions arose in my shaking body as opposing desires were at war. Should I run from the horror *or* turn to love? Out loud, I said to my mirror image, "I'm in."

DOI: 10.4324/9781003386339-9

In this chapter, I describe and illustrate the power of building a mutual aid community based on the emerging needs of a group. A group is compiled by many unique individuals. Sometimes the only commonality in our groups was a shared HIV diagnosis. The diversity of group composition contributes to the unique resources that are available to all from a mutual aid perspective. The contributions of an individual will often mobilize the group forward towards its unfolding purpose. Therefore, I begin this chapter with a study of one individual's experience of receiving an HIV diagnosis in the first known decade of AIDS. Greg Fowler discovered he was HIV positive in 1988, and recorded his experiences in a journal that he graciously has shared with us. The entries in Greg's journal illustrate the immediacy of his unique personal experiences. At the same time, certain themes about Greg's existential and physical concerns resonated with many other individuals who were also HIV positive, illustrated below.

The section entitled "A Mutual Aid Approach to Group and Community Practice" summarizes the basic principles of psychodrama theory and practice, from which we established an ethos of mutual aid that is instrumental in creating a cohesive climate for healing and social change. I illustrate the veracity of the psychodramatic method with a session I conducted with Lucas Harris, the co-founder of Project Quest. The tenderness of Lucas's drama opened the group to new dimensions of grief, and empowerment in the face of death. The drama also demonstrates how essential a heuristic approach is in a process-oriented group.

Because much of our work in community building included residential retreats, the chapter also follows the unfolding process of a single AIDS retreat. The retreat began with a sudden, horrific, and life-threatening experience for one of our participants. I describe how the group responded to the horror of this event, and how we as group leaders responded to a challenging group process. Greg would play an important role, with others, by challenging my trustworthiness as an outsider. Central themes about trust, vulnerability, dependency, desire, and how to love arose.

The final section explores the flexibility of dual-role relationships that necessarily emerge in times of collective crises. Relationships develop out of the concrete realities of everyday life. Greg, for example, would become one of my closest family friends, and formed unique intimate relationships with Graham and Lusijah that have endured to the present day.

Becoming HIV Positive: Greg Fowler's Story

Greg Fowler has graciously shared key sections of his personal journal describing the first weeks following his HIV diagnosis in 1988. I select sections from two journal entries and discuss salient themes that emerged following each entry.

Greg: April 22, 1988

On Monday, I turned thirty years old. It's supposed to be one of those traumatic experiences, right? People at work must have thought I was taking it particularly bad. Who could I talk to? Was there anyone who could understand – when you get to the point that you feel your whole life had ended....and the mere fact of turning thirty is the least important thing you can think of.

When I went into Dr. P's office that day, what did I expect? To be honest, I was prepared for the worst. I felt I knew my body, and the swollen lymph nodes I knew were indicative of a much larger problem. .....The answer came easy as I walked through the door. All it took was a simple quip on his part: "We do not have good news for modern man." And he again expressed his surprise that the test was positive...but of course this was irrelevant. And the complications began to set in.

How complicated my life would become. The big question of confidentiality. How to deal with insurance, with my job, with my family...with the whole damn rest of my life. And the anger...the anger I felt towards the people who had used me when I had first come out. The anger towards myself...for letting myself and my family down. For my life being a failure. The ultimate failure, and I would die. The thought of death did not bother me as much as the failure, and the loss of faith in the world around me and the people I had known in my life. And the sadness in my attempt of having some hope in a god which I had tried to believe in, and the anger towards him, first, for making me gay, and then for killing me for it. And the bottomless disappointment...for living my whole life, and giving the ultimate sacrifice, my life, just for the chance of finding someone who could, who might love me, and having failed in this. And I did not want to live.

How to describe for someone who has never been through this? For all of my life, even when things had seemed the most hopeless, even when I thought I had nothing left and even toyed with the idea of suicide, I still felt I had control. CONTROL. I could not find love, and sometimes not even friendship. I often failed at things I had attempted. But deep down inside, I felt I always had some control left. Now there was nothing left. I was totally alone, as I had been most of my life, but this time I did not even have myself to depend on. I had lost myself and all meaning and control over my existence. I was never so helpless.

At home, in the relative safety of my aloneness, and the total aloneness of it, everything broke loose. I laid in the grass of my backyard, yelling, and screaming out of control. I had lost everything. Nothing was left. There was no hope, no life. Everything had conquered my being. There is no way to describe it. No way.

GB Fowler

Greg was utterly seized by a reality that was impossible to grasp. He was now living in the epicenter of his own death's reality as a young man. His ability to think rationally had contributed to his success as an accountant, but now he had lost control of many things, most importantly his own body. He could not think of the trajectory of his life going forward. He was lost to himself. *"Everything has conquered my being."*

During Greg's anguish (and I weep reading his words) he confesses that *all he desired, has ever desired, is love and to be loved, a desire he now feels is insurmountably and cruelly crushed by an unfair fate.* Greg rages at himself for "letting himself down" for contracting the virus in the first place, and towards those who had emotionally and physically exploited his vulnerability when he first came out. He rages at himself for now bearing another stain (AIDS in addition to being gay) and fears further alienation from his family and broader social world.

In the first wave of grief, we can see how his own terrible shame for being fallible takes hold, a failure he carries with him because of earlier implied deprivations. The shame-stain of being gay, his rage at god (he used lower case g, already a diminished god in his mind) for making him so, and who then is ruthlessly "killing him" with AIDS.

Greg: April 25, 1988

Time heals many things. You go into the fire, and then you come out again, but are you the same? Last Monday night, with the depression I felt, and the many considerations...like that of being a martyr, and keeping the pain to myself, I did tell my sister. We sat upon the couch for a long while, slowly talking of the many ways it would affect us. Her, telling me how unfair it was. Me, responding by asking what is fair? She would rub my hair, as a mother would a child...comforting the moment, knowing that the future would be many unanswered questions.

Tuesday morning, trying to hold the pieces of the puzzle, of my life together as it starts to fall apart faster than I can put it back together. Coming to the realization, that I've never had before – that I cannot make it alone. By nine o'clock that morning, I knew I had to call someone before I totally disintegrated. I had been given the number of a P H by Dr. P. Dr. P. had described P.H. and I half-way knew who he was because he was a regular habitual Y goer like me. So, I called, introducing myself by telling him I didn't know why I was calling, but only that I know I couldn't make it by myself. Just having someone to listen to me....

The attitude that no one really cares about each other in the gay world, so who was this strange creature called P H. That night, P H called me on the phone, and we talked a long while. I began to feel more comfortable, and that maybe I could control things...maybe I could experience what happiness was again.

GB Fowler

Half ruined from grief and rage while also consumed with what now seemed like an impossible desire to live *with* AIDS, Greg is visited by a radical new thought: "I know I couldn't make it by myself." We feel his ongoing struggle to either fall back on his reliance to isolatively self-care *or* alternatively take the terrifying risk of asking for help. Asking for help would expose him to the possibility of further rejection, abandonment, and exploitation. Who of us is not familiar with this fundamental struggle, now magnified by a deadly disease?

In a leap of faith beyond the conserves of who he used to be, Greg shares his diagnosis with his sister. The tenderness of this passage burns through the page. When there is nothing to say, her fingers express love in a timeless language. The holder is also held, as together they contemplate an unknown and terrifying future. In moments such these, we are not alone. But whom could he now trust in the gay community or anywhere else? Greg made a reference to a cultural bias regarding the superficiality of the gay community (alluded to in the first entry) because of his experiences of being sexually and emotionally exploited by other gay men. He was afraid to give himself over again. He took the risk and made a call to a new therapist, giving him a *sense of control* again, where he could begin to imagine the possibility of having a life worth living with AIDS and not be alone.

Greg refers to a number of human themes about his desire to care and be cared for. In the psychodrama and the AIDS retreat discussed below, we will see how centrally shared the needs for mutuality and intimate connection become. Recall the work of physician and evolutionary sociologist Nicholas Christakis (2019), discussed in Chapter 1. Christakis holds the view that we are innately equipped as a species to band together, live cooperatively with each other, recognize uniqueness, show kindness, love, and reciprocity in our relationships, learn socially, and teach what we know. How we care for each other, in other words, is at least partially encoded in our genes, and fundamental to building to what he calls "good" societies. How some groups coalesce into societies that uphold these innate sensibilities is the topic of the next section. There, I re-introduce basic principles of group psychology.

A Mutual Aid Approach to Group and Community Psychology

Graham, Lusijah, and I co-led many local groups and residential therapy retreats together as the Quest community was forming. While our clinical orientations were diverse, each of us had psychodrama training in common. We believe this contributed to our capacity to develop a mutual aid ethos and shared belief in the healing power of group psychotherapy. In the first two decades of AIDS, there was little research within mainstream mental health about plague or collective trauma, group psychotherapy, or trauma therapy. While we also worked with developmental trauma that preceded an AIDS diagnosis, our growing edge as clinicians was in developing new ways of understanding and working with plague trauma as it affected and/or impaired the individual and/or group's capacity to live fully into death or life's possibility.

I was in the early stages of becoming a Jungian analyst, and was therefore integrating aspects of Jungian psychology into my work with groups.[1] Jungian psychotherapy (analytical psychology) is directed from our engagement with our depths (psyche), in a process of self-development called individuation. This process can be traced in turning points, or moments of change, facilitated by the emergence of universal (archetypal) themes, patterns, and/or symbols.[2] My Jungian analysis with Bob Stuckey was a life-line throughout, as I kept opening to others, to love, to grief, the unknown, my mind, my own depths and opacities. Opening to radical love has altered my life. The capacity to self-reflect is a form of self-care from which authentic mutuality is possible. In other words, our ability to support each other in co-leadership, and in mutual aid cultures, is determined by our self-reflective capacity that is nurtured by our own psychotherapy (or analysis), spiritual practices, and/or other forms of self-care that become acutely crucial in a sustained crisis.

Psychoanalysis (in general) does not apply its theories and methods to groups or collectives, or to their developmental processes. Nevertheless, in this vacuum, I began to more acutely notice how universal themes emerged in our groups, mobilized by the inner forces of the group as a whole and often through the therapy work of an individual. Jacob Levey Moreno, the founder of group psychotherapy, referred to these inner forces as the dynamic interchange between co-unconscious and co-conscious processes that are always already at play in every group meeting. I noticed that when these themes are recognized and engaged, they facilitate a group's individuation, or rather guide a transformative process towards its unfolding purpose. I further illustrate how universal themes emerge in the group process in the next section and in Chapter 9.

On a meta-level, the development of a cohesive Quest community and eventual AIDS clinic in 1989 was a liberatory outcome of community individuation amidst a broader, cross-cultural, national, and global gay rights and AIDS activist movement in response to dominating psychosocial and geopolitical factors that sought to invisiblize the reality. In other words, the synchronistic vertex from which Quest emerged needs to be understood in the polarizing yet revolutionary context of AIDS activism.

Mutual aid practices enhance group cohesion and the group's natural tendency to develop and share their depths. These practices draw on its members' strengths, ways of knowing, shared sense of security, and purpose. Embracing a mutual aid approach to group leadership meant that we retained a soft hierarchical stance in group work. Power (influence), responsibility, and resources are shared. Individual concerns are identified and attended to within an egalitarian process. Nobody is left behind. We support inter- and intra-connection (self to self and self to other) through various sociometric and psychodramatic techniques that support social bonding, build resilience, and inspire social coop-eration. Group cohesion is furthered still by a personal desire to survive and the chaotic urge to live fully that lies at the root of personal and collective agency. Building a relationship with our depths (self to self) supports a more authentic and maturing capacity to care for and receive care from others.

Our depth-psychological orientations and shared psychodrama training guided us as we attempted to understand and interpret what was happening with the group as a whole while also tracking individual dynamics. Our formative group history or family-of-origin experiences shape how individuals function in groups. Therefore, we observed and worked with projective processes and trans-ference phenomena (including trans-generational influences) that inevitably arose and impeded self and group development, using a variety of psychodra-matic action techniques including sociometric and sociodramatic explorations.

Sociometry, sociodrama, psychodrama, and group psychotherapy are the four branches of study one must master to become a certified psychodrama practi-tioner (Certified Practitioner) or trainer (Trainer, Educator, and Practitioner) of psychodrama. Sociometry is a qualitative method and action technique invented by Romanian-born American psychiatrist Jacob Levy Moreno (in the 1930s), de-signed for measuring the social interrelationships of a group.[3] I discuss Moreno at some length in Chapter 3 and 9. We regularly used sociometric methods in action to unmask the individual and group dynamics that shaped the choices participants made with each other. Sociometry can also reveal the alliances, hid-den beliefs, and forbidden agendas at play that divide a group or alternatively enhance cohesion (Williams, 1991, pp. 127–128).

Each person holds a unique subjective position that contributes to how a group functions and therefore has something to teach the group about itself. For example, there is almost always an isolate in a group. The isolate, in sociometric theory, is the least socially connected to others on various criteria. This is in contrast to other group members who are more socially connected.[4] There are many reasons that isolates exist in group life, and few of us can say that we have not been an isolate in a group situation. Modeling inclusivity while recognizing diversity is a crucial function for any group leader living within a differentiated humanity. Also, exploring the psychodynamic mechanisms that contribute to in-dividual isolation and how a group may collude with these dynamics is a regular feature of group therapy.

Psychodrama theory and practice was founded on egalitarian principles. Briefly stated here, Moreno (1889–1974) argued throughout his life that the in-dividual's access to spontaneity and creativity was a key component to a pos-sibility of living fully in a diverse world. On this point he elaborated:

If there is any primary principle in the mental and social universe, it is found in the twin concept [of spontaneity and creativity] which has its most tangi-ble reality in the interplay between person and person, between person and

things, between person and work, between society and society, between society and the whole of mankind, between mankind and the physical world
around it.

(Moreno, 1955, p. 105)

We can quickly see from this emblematic quotation that Moreno, in contrast
to most traditional psychotherapy and psychoanalytic approaches, viewed the
individual as a psyche/social being. The individual is co-created by one's em-
beddedness in the concrete and social world. Creativity is a response to a need
for change that arises from an individual in an effort to respond in a novel way
to a new situation or an adequate way to a familiar one (Moreno, 1946, pp. 50,
134). Spontaneity is not a random or a chance response to a dilemma posed, but
a "catalyzer" from which creative action arises (Moreno, 1955, p. 105).[5]

Moreno believed in and advocated for the healing power of group processes
because he observed that group members could be healing agents for each other
if their barriers to creativity could be worked through. His therapeutic methods
allowed for "sociometric explorations" that could enhance mutual connectivity
and group cohesion. This can be achieved by examining the group's shadow
(the unconscious dynamics), discovered by exploring projective processes that
impair singular and collective creative possibilities (Ulon & Brooks, 2018). The
psychodramatic method is an action method that brings alive the stories and/or
concerns of the protagonist by using the group members as supportive agents.

Psychodrama is often called *a rehearsal for living.* Extending Jung into
group psychology, I continually notice that we often tap into universal human
processes that are taking place in the personality of the individual, activated in
depth group work. What arises within the individual may also reflect moments of
change or transformative turning points in the group as a whole. These processes
are facilitated by the appearance of archetypal patterns, collective themes, or
symbols. In what follows, I illustrate how death became a transformative turning
point for the whole group as the protagonist enacted a scene depicting his death
and how he wanted to be cared for through it.

Psychodrama Illustrated

Lucas Harris was the co-founder of Project Quest. His health was beginning to
rapidly fail when he attended this retreat in the mid-1990s. Anti-viral cocktails
(HAART) would not be released until the following year (unbeknownst to us)
so death was imminent for many in that room. Nevertheless, Lucas was a physically striking man—fiery and trickster like in his often provocative and shockingly direct manner, not bothering with the banality of nuanced conversation.[6]

The psychodramatic session began when Lucas walked to the center of the
room, non-verbally identifying that he was putting himself forward as a protagonist. Nobody else came forward. After a brief silence, *Lucas declared that*

he wanted to create (psychodramatically) *the scene of his own death* and that he wanted me to direct him. With co-leadership, the protagonist can choose the person they want to direct their psychodramatic process. I had not yet directed a protagonist's death scene, and certainly not the death scene of someone who was my friend, and a friend of my family, and the honor washed over me. In one evanescent moment, Lucas's psychodrama ushered many of us into the living sacred space of high ceremony—a ceremony that would speak to many in that room because of his courage to face his own death directly, challenging each of us to hold this fundamental truth ourselves, *with him.*

Lucas went about creating the scene of his death, using props to concretize the space. He constructed his bed, noted the time of day, and identified who he wanted to be in the room of his death chamber. I was shaken and deeply moved when he declared that he wanted me to actually *be with him* during his dying time and death. "Can you do this for me," he earnestly asked, "direct my drama and be in it, too? And sit with me through my death?" His tender and earnest gaze met mine as "his spirit touched my body," in the words of the Sufi poet Rumi.[7] I surrendered to the task, and to him. I knew that guiding a ritual where we all bore witness to what he needed would require sustained emotional engagement from all of us. He was asking us to *turn towards a truth, with him ... a truth that was shared* because many in that room were hinging between life and imminent death, and all of us are mortal. He was also asking me to actually be there with him (and others) in his actual dying time.

"Yes," I said, looking directly into his dark eyes. "But you will need to choose an auxiliary to play me in the drama. I cannot direct and play another role at the same time. And, yes, my friend, I will be with you in real time when it comes."[8] We locked eyes. He nodded. Such a tender moment. He then chose somebody from the group to play "Robin," placing them on the left side of the death bed prop. He identified several other people and carefully placed auxiliary role players (or actual people if they were present) where he wanted them in his death chamber. Through a series of role reversals, Lucas showed his auxiliaries *in action* how he specified what he wanted to hear from each of us—including silence. He also demonstrated in action the kinds of touch he wanted, including the tender bathing of his corpse. I can barely type the words to describe the tenderness of this scene.

Finally, Lucas chose someone in the room to role play himself. The auxiliary playing "Lucas" placed himself in the bed accordingly. Standing with Lucas on the perimeter of the staged space, I asked the auxiliaries to play back the scene as he had shown them. We observed the auxiliary Lucas, receiving specified care through his final breath, followed by the psychodramatic bathing of his dead body. The room was very quiet, in full attentive mode except for one or two who appeared to be sleeping. Some were quietly crying. After a while, I asked: "How is this for you?" He was riveted, nodded, and said he wanted to see it played out again. While the scene was playing out again, I asked him if he wanted to role reverse with the person playing his part for the experience of it, or was this enough? He reflected, and then moved towards his fantasy death bed.

Lucas was weak from illness and nearly collapsed while situating himself in the staged death bed, but appeared to be buoyed by the profoundness of what was unfolding. I then instructed the auxiliaries to, one at a time, play out their roles as given them by Lucas. For a moment, he quietly received the ministrations from his mock death chamber. *Suddenly*, he rose from the scene and awkwardly joined me on the perimeter. "I am not dead yet," he dramatically retorted, flashing a trickster smile and head twist. Gut-releasing laughter filled the room. We had come close to the life/death membrane, and it was a relief to only be rehearsing for death at the moment.

The poignancy of this drama is beyond description, and I will remember it for the rest of my life. I recall the late afternoon lighting of the scene as the winter sun slowly faded. There was such a quiet respect in the room, alongside heart-wrenching tears and break-out wicked humor. Joy can accompany profound grief in the uncanniest ways—one of the miracles of psychodramatic work when a whole group becomes enlivened with the protagonist and carries the drama into another transformative dimension.

Following the drama, Lucas returned to the group circle and collapsed in another group member's arms as we shifted into what we call the "sharing phase." Sharing after an enactment allows group members to relay their personal experience, either from a role that they played in the drama and/or as an audience member from the sidelines. Comments are not directed to the protagonist, who often is still in an altered state, metabolizing their experience. Personal sharing is directly related to the individual's personal experience and sometimes may warm them up to their own psychodrama. We all knew that Lucas was dying. He would actually die the following spring, and was accompanied, for the most part, as he had envisioned it.[9]

Collective Loss and Mourning

Paul Attinello, a Jungian analyst and long-term survivor of AIDS, recalled his experience during the early days of AIDS. Analysts (and I add other clinicians of any orientation), he said, are not adequately trained to be with the material or psychical realities of dying or death with our patients, then or now (Attinello, 2023). This was especially evidenced in the COVID-19 pandemic.

Erik Goodwyn, psychiatrist and Jungian scholar, conducted an interdisciplinary analysis of mourning and complicated grief that arises when one is not able to move through a mourning process. Goodwyn (2015) outlines a composite of characteristics across cultures that he suggests aids in a mourning process. In brief, these basic elements include providing a cultural container for raw emotionality to be situated in a culturally defined context; recognition of the vulnerability of bereaved and community; creating a framework to reframe and reorganize the relationship between the bereaved and deceased; employing methods to physically enact, contain, and channel emotional expression in culturally specific ways; and finally employing methods to integrate the death into a coherent narrative compatible with surrounding belief systems. Goodwyn further characterizes an almost absolute absence of care that facilitates a mourning process as described above in the United States today (2015, pp. 259–261).

Mourning is a natural response to loss and cannot happen in isolation. We need each other so that we may mourn through whatever cultural traditions or practices we have. Liberation psychologist Ignacio Martín-Baró stressed the importance of recovering historical cultural memory amidst collective trauma. Remembering our traditions, culture, and ancestorial heritage provides a container through which we may process our grief in the service of liberation from the socio-cultural induced fatalism so that we can *take hold of our own fate* (Martín-Baró, 1994, p. 30). Reconfiguring our core identity and sense of purpose going forward relies on the ability to creatively retain a deepening sense of who we are, in the face of massive disorientation. In the absence of adequate traditions, however, community healing practices, such as Lucas created in his psychodrama, can be co-created in mutual aid–oriented groups as we become healing agents for each other.

Mind–body medicine supports the psycho/spiritual embodied experiences that emerge in group practice. Our approaches were diverse and included psychodynamically informed traditions, group psychotherapy, psychodrama, sociometry, sociodrama, ceremony/ritual building, art-making, telling and listening to one's story, hypnotic visualization, dream work, expressive arts, body-oriented therapies (acupuncture, yoga, exercise, sweat lodges, erotic dance), and other integrative medicines (Indigenous, nature, food and plant medicines, allopathic, and traditional). Adapting a heuristic approach is leavened by the practitioner who can access other knowledge systems, whatever they are.

A heuristic approach problem-solves through practice and experience rather than working *exclusively* with an already formulated theory, often in collaboration with other group leaders, and always following the emerging needs of the group and individual. This does not mean we throw out all theories of mind and totally rely on creative immersion in the work. When traditional theories are not relevant to the situation at hand, we organically create new ways of being and thinking about what is happening *in situ*. We improvise, in other words becoming an instrument of a process, with the group members, which is always mysterious, uncertain, anxiety provoking, and sometimes transformative.

The qualities that support a heuristic approach begin with the capacity to follow closely what is needed by group members. Following the emerging needs of the group participants is a form of mutuality that invites co-transparency, self-revelation, cultivates the expression of care, group cohesion, individuality, and what is universal in the human experience. I summarize these qualities below:

1. *Fosters inclusivity* through welcoming differences of all kinds while holding a clear "frame." The frame attends to time parameters; follows the values of mutual aid and care but not to the exclusion of self-care; welcomes through warmth; speaks well of others; is generous, consistent, and curious about others and what they need; retains a sense of humor.
2. *Follows the needs of group members* by allowing space for individual discovery; listens carefully; is humble, patient, and open to influence; flexible in changing a direction.
3. *Supports new ideas, desires, and needs of individuals and the group as whole*: builds trust by following through in group decisions and purpose; is reliable; attends to what is needed in the community; fosters a decision-making process by encouraging new forms of leadership rising in the group; acknowledges one's limitations and gaps of knowing.
4. *Clarity in communication*: vulnerable when moved; appropriately transparent; willing to engage the uncertain and what can be learned from difficult situations and models this stance; articulates as clearly, directly, and concisely as possible while responding to group needs.
5. *Thinking on one's feet in a fast changing or perplexing situation*: engages group wisdom and/or that of a colleague, co-leader, and group member; models problem-solving with co-leaders at times during group sessions; changes mind when necessary and can step back and change directions (co-leadership stepping in, new emerging need from the group etc.); willingness to be innovative and creative if methodology is failing.

The group is only a whole, if we consider the plurality from which universal themes of the human condition emerge. The very human themes Greg Fowler described in his journal entry above, such as needing to be loved and cared for upon receiving an HIV diagnosis, give us insight into the psychodrama retreat that follows. The following section illustrates further how crucial the capacity of thinking and feeling on one's feet really is.

One AIDS Retreat Discussed and Illustrated

I start with a vignette:

Lusijah, Graham, and I were co-leading a psychodrama retreat on Orcas Island in the early 1990s. Twenty-nine participants living with AIDS attended this retreat, many of whom did not know each other. During the first night, one of the participants, who I will refer to as "Connie," started to menstruate and the blood flowed out of her body for hours onto her clothing, her bedding, and the mattress, pooling onto the floor where we found her the next morning. Whomever first saw her (nobody remembers now) encountered what looked like a horrific crime scene. On first sight, she looked dead although she was in a coma from blood loss. The pungent mineral scent of her blood lingered in the dark, still room. Engaging Connie's blood and what that foretold catapulted us into another dimension of time or timelessness. Quite suddenly, many group members lunged wordlessly into collective action. I can only describe it as a timeless whoosh where Connie was now being carried out of her dank room on her bloody mattress on the shoulders of many participants towards a van that would take her to a hospital off island. She looked like Mantegna's image of the dead Christ, yet she was still breathing. Greg Carrigan describes the moment this way: "We could all see our own death then and it was at the same time so healing because we were all lifting her on her mattress, over us … she floated over the top of us" (Brooks, 2022, pp. 45–46). During this somber procession, Jesse Isaac started playing a flute from the porch of the main house. Long sorrowful notes accompanied them all the way to the van. We watched Lusijah and Wasaka pull away with Connie safely harbored in fresh blankets towards her fate. What I remember next was that Graham and I were now seated on a couch in the main house holding hands crazed with shock and horror, profoundly uncertain about what would happen next. The group was gathering for the first session of a shattered day. "Are you ready?" I asked Graham. He nodded slowly. "Such a tender moment." We then stood up and moved into "a fierce eddy of intelligible forces that were swirling around and through us" (revised Brooks, 2018, 2022).[10]

Connie's bleeding out ignited in a flashpoint moment, when group members *suddenly and collectively* lifted Connie up, on her bloody mattress, and carried her to the van to save her life. Transformative moments like this one are living expressions of mutual aid and group cohesion.

Connie was a First Nation woman, in a group of gay men who were also living with AIDS. Although Lusijah (group leader) and Wasaka Borgelt (ally) knew her well, Connie was a social isolate because she was the only woman participant in an otherwise all gay male group. Furthermore, the vicerality of her menstrual blood highlighted her difference and, in Jungian parlance, constelled a collective theme of abject vulnerability, helplessness, and dependency. Recall the sociometric principle that views the isolate in the group as one who has the most to teach the group about itself. Connie's differences were transcended when her helplessness opened each of us to a shared truth about our *own* vulnerability, as little animals beyond the *puniverse* of the individual.[11] As Graham Harriman stated it: "This very dynamic of inclusivity, based on the perception that *we all are vulnerable*, led to a sense of collective empowerment that characterizes HIV advocacy to this day" (personal conversation, April 18, 2020). In the following section, I describe how the trauma of Connie's near-death experience deepened the group therapy sessions that followed. I am interested in demonstrating how a universal process contributes to the transformative process of the whole group.

"What Do You Do with a Man If You Aren't Fucking Him?"

Graham and I were leading the session that immediately followed Connie's departure to the hospital off island, in the van driven by Lusijah and Wasaka. As described in the vignette above, Graham and I were sitting on a couch together, in a room with everybody else. The session began. Following a long silence, participant Greg Fowler suddenly stood up and directly addressed me with the full force of his person. His body was frail from weight loss, but his voice was fierce and fiery. *"What do you know about AIDS, or my life, you with your family in that big house on the hill, driving an all-wheel-drive mini-van?"* I met Greg for the first time during this retreat and his sudden encounter caught me utterly off guard. His wildly disarranged thick dark hair and dark penetrating eyes strangely pulled me out of myself towards him. I was pulled in between the two of us, now vulnerable to whatever would happen next. I was stunned and red-faced, ashamed. "How dare I," he was asking me, "come into our lives, his life … like I knew anything about our experience."

Indeed, why should he blindly trust me? He was right. I did not know him. We did not know each other. I had led a number of HIV retreats, but I was not gay, not HIV positive and lived in a white hetero bubble, unsullied personally by the virus. Both of us were flushed and trembling. I met his harsh gaze with soft intensity. I said something like this: "I don't know anything about your life, Greg, or what it is like living with AIDS or being gay. You are right. I hope you will tell me." I was trembling and raw faced. The room was entirely silent. We sat there for a while, steadily holding eye contact, and then he looked away. Enough for now.

Retrospectively, I suspect that Greg was in part emboldened because he already trusted Graham. Graham is gay, living with AIDS, and they knew each other from other contexts. Working with Graham gave me accountability because of these alliances, but I had to stand on the virtue of my own humanity. The second point I would like to make is that the poignancy of Greg's challenge likely grew out of his own desire for intimacy, stimulated by the group's expression of care for Connie, and thus for each other. Put another way, the group was banding together following Connie's ordeal, although this was never directly expressed at this time. If the group climate encourages personal honesty, and the therapists can receive such a challenging address, participants are more likely to step forward and risk revealing what is on their mind and in their heart. Psyche erupts. Also, once the authenticity and capability of the group leader is established, then individuals in the group may feel freer to explore their interpersonal relationships with each other, in addition to sharing their personal material.

Greg's encounter with me was intimate and real. His AIDS status had already emotionally and physically exposed *him* to *me*, but until he challenged me, *I had not yet revealed my own vulnerability as a person to him or the others.* If Greg was going to be able to join, or make full use of, the group he needed to establish that I could be trusted. I too needed to be vulnerable and sincere about my limitations, in a caring, human, *mutual exchange*. The basis of this exchange required that we meet each other, face to face, and be changed by it.

Following this encounter, there was a prolonged silence in the room of 27 or so participants. Graham and I waited. Then, somebody I will call "Doug" asked a rhetorical question that deepened and refined the course of the retreat. "*What do you do with a man if you aren't fucking him?*" The entire room exploded in anxious laughter—a form of unspoken solidarity and relief. As we worked with Doug further, he began to clarify what was behind his initial question that may be rhetorically summarized this way: "*How can I be seen or see another gay man as anything other than a sexual object not to be trusted?*" or "*Can a gay man value anything else about me other than my asshole?*" and, if so, "*What do you value about me?*" "*How can I relate to you and you to me, if not as a sexual object?*" Ultimately, these concerns led to: "*What is friendship?*" and "*How can I be a friend?*"

We can trace the turning points within the group's process that were activated by a series of encounters, that in turn facilitated the transformation of the group as a whole towards a common purpose. Connie's near-death experience and the group's spontaneous collective response to *save her life* mobilized the archetypal theme of human desire to love and be loved, and for the expression of radical love in the face of its impossibility. This was followed by Greg's encounter with me, demanding a mutual exchange that illustrated how trust can be established so that mutuality can exist. The theme of mutual respect mobilized Doug's expressed desire to have intimate friendships and his despair about how mutual care is achieved. The rest of the retreat continued to focus on this theme that included exploring individual barriers to intimacy that were largely related to socialization wounds, homophobia, earlier family-of-origin traumas, breaches of trust, and societal degradation.

Later that night, Lusijah and Wasaka returned from the mainland hospital where Connie was being treated. Her life had been saved for now. Together, we designed a skills development program for establishing and maintaining friendships right there, on the spot. This program would extend into the next year and beyond. Support groups were formed, and plans were made for therapist follow-up with each support group throughout the year.

Dual Roles in an Egalitarian Community of Care

As clinicians, we expanded *the therapeutic stage to life as it is lived and where it is lived*, not contained to an office, as the times called for that. Below, I discuss how dual roles enrichened my life and contributed to many mutual exchanges "across borders."

I had many dual roles with Quest community members, such as attending a commitment ceremony where my son was a flower boy, hospital visits, being with a person through dying and death's passage, attending sweat lodge ceremonies, co-leading a presentation at a conference, delivering extra HIV drugs (after a patient died) to the underground pipeline for distribution to those in need, home visits of all kinds, sharing and making art, purchasing art, Lucas cutting my son's hair, receiving or giving gifts, helping and being helped moving households, cooking together, giving and receiving emotional support, guitar lessons for my son, hiring a nanny for my son, climbing mountains together, sharing a tent, sharing holidays, attending various cultural functions, and inviting Quest members to my wedding, my son's eagle scout ceremony, my son's wedding, and so on. As time wore on, I became friends with some of the community members and continue to share key moments in life with them to this day.

My relationship with Greg Fowler, for example, grew into a lifelong friendship. In the late 1990s Greg asked me if I would help him organize a mountaineering branch of what was called *Team Quest*. He said I was better at organizing groups and if I helped him, he would teach me how to climb above the timberline. Team Quest was created by Ken Ballard in the mid-1990s as an adjunct program in Project Quest that provided athletic activities for those living with HIV/AIDS and other life-threatening conditions. Brice Winters was a team manager of one of Team Quest's soft ball teams, not having the strength to actually play the game but able to support the team (Dudley, 1999, *Oregonian*, March 5). Player Paul Moore had a pick line in for a while. As participant (softball and climbing team) Tad Williams stated it: "Team Quest welcomes everyone and anyone ... All skill levels can come and play ... that makes it a nonthreatening way for people to get out and have fun and meet people" (Ibid.).

I agreed to collaborate with Greg in building a mountaineering arm of Team Quest. Together with many others, we hiked, backpacked, and climbed many mountains. Greg described how the dream of climbing became a central motivation that would carry him beyond the immediate limitations of severe illness in an article for *Oregon and S.W. Washington HIV Positive Newsletter* prior to our first major climb. He wrote:

I've been asked why someone with AIDS would want to climb a mountain. Aren't there enough things to deal with, right? But maybe that's just it. With so many things to deal with, climbing a mountain can seem like a good alternative. I remember lying in bed three years ago after my move to Portland. I'd just gone through PCP followed by Aspergillosis. I would focus myself away from my illness to the peak of Mt Hood rising in the distant horizon. The thought of climbing the mountain was one of the motivations that could carry me beyond my present limitations. That thought became the impetus for my continued health and well-being. It was the thing that got me up in the morning, to down the necessary pills, eat a good breakfast, and if I felt good enough, to go to the gym. By the next summer, even though my T-cells were

still below 50, I managed to wheeze my way up to the summit of Mt Hood.
That, more than anything else, reaffirmed my commitment to life.

(Fowler, 1999)

The above passage illustrates what McGonigal describes as choosing to see the
"upside of adversity" (2015, p. 201). She concludes that such a stance requires
an ability to notice the good as you cope with things that are difficult in such a
way that does not just improve physical health, but can also protect one against
depression and strengthen relationships (Ibid., pp. 202–203). Embracing the upside of adversity does not mean disavowing what is adverse. In this model, one
calls on a capacity to hold a tension between a raw truth of AIDS and the possibilities for a life worth living without splitting into fundamentalist extremes:
Having AIDS sucks *or* I am a divine being of light. Both are real.

Greg's capacity to see the upside of adversity allowed him to believe that
mountaineering within a team would potentially assist others to also cope with
their diagnosis, by living fully with what is physically possible *now.* Fourteen
people committed to climbing Mt. Rainier the first time over the ensuing seven
months with only one person dropping out. Our team consisted of ten men and
three women, each facing a variety of challenges including HIV/AIDS and a heart
transplant. We had professional guides who required that each of us qualify prior to
our ascent. Two climbers, Casey Merideth and Aaron Hornstein, gloriously summited Rainier that day. Three years prior, Aaron, 32 years old, was sent home to
die but the antiviral cocktail he was given started working and he "came back from
the brink" (Dudley, 1999, *Oregonian*, March 5, August 9). Casey was later quoted
(on a plaque) saying that: "The climb is a metaphor for life itself … lofty summits,
teamwork, exertion, careful direction and execution, stage setting and completion." Ken Ballard describes the thrill of their return this way. "There was such a
sense of triumph, knowing what they went through, not just on the mountain, but
everything it took to get there" (Boulé, 1999, *Oregonian*, August 9, August 15).

Greg Fowler produced a YouTube video of a second Mt. Rainier climb in
July 2002 with Christopher Carloss as the videographer. Chris carried a heavy
camera in addition to his climbing gear without a grumble. In a later Mt. Rainier
climb, Saskia Von Micholovski and Mary Gilsen-Mendel guided us for free and/
or donation to pay for the food they provided. Saskia had previously guided us
on the Mt. Baker climb in 2000. Other Team Quest allies such as Jim O'Hearn,
a physician, Jeffrey Burdick, and Deb Gruber joined this expedition.[12] On my
way to the trailhead, I visited Brice Winters at the VA, having heard he was in
an acute health crisis. When I asked him if he wanted me to stay with him, he
looked into me with his blue eyes and told me to go. "I'll be with you every step
of the way." By this he meant all of us. We learned of Brice's death as we were
loading up our packs in the parking lot of White River Campground. Brice had
given us his blessing. Coming down from the climb, we were met at Glacier
Basin campground by two of his friends, Shellie Barich and Colleen Groll, who

brought us cold beer to celebrate his life. Brice was a recovering alcoholic and would have appreciated the irony.

Other climbs organized by Team Quest included Mt. St. Helens, WA (1997); Mt. Baker, WA (2000); Mt. St. Helens, WA, Middle Sister, OR (2002); Mt. Hood, OR, Mt Adams, WA, and Mt. Rainier, WA (2002); Kilimanjaro, Tanzania, Africa (2003); Mt. Adams, WA (2004); South Sister and Broken Top, OR (2005). Christopher Carloss also produced another YouTube video of the Kilimanjaro climb entitled: Kilimanjaro: *Climb for Life*. Greg co-edited the documentary revealing the challenges encountered in the expedition of living with HIV/AIDS. Greg became the first American person living with AIDS to have summited Kilimanjaro.

AIDS would become a traumatizing *and* a revolutionary flash point for the gay rights movement and HIV/AIDS activism across the globe, as it had become in our town. Quest was a sparkling light in a vast sky of revolution. Lessons learned from grassroots HIV/gay advocacy movements show us how mutual aid communities, in their various forms, supported the empowerment of disenfranchised persons across the land in the face of impossible hope (Halkitis, 2015; France, 2016; Schulman, 2021).[13]

Notes

1 I discuss this in more detail in Chapter 9 of this book, and also from a psychoanalytic perspective in *Psychoanalysis, Catastrophe and Social Change* (Brooks, 2022).
2 This process of individuation continues to be the heart of analytical psychology. Jung's attempt to map this process in its universal form is the reason behind his interest in alchemy, mythology (the hero's journey), and spiritual traditions because traces of this process can be found in all of these fields.
3 Moreno defined sociometry as "the mathematical study of psychological properties of populations, the experimental technique of and the results obtained by application of quantitative methods" (Moreno, 1953, pp. 15–16).
4 Sometimes an individual does not have any social connections to others in the group because they are a new group member. An isolate may already be an established member of the group but may have not established mutual connections with other group members. These may be hidden or unconscious forces at play but can be revealed in sociometric explorations. Alterity, or otherness that always and dynamically exist within groups may be bound to perceived and threatening differences such as gender, sexual orientation, race, educational/psychological/socio-economic status, popularity, or whatever is valued as attractive that the isolate does not hold.
5 Spontaneity arises from the readiness of the subject to respond adequately to a situation in the moment (Ibid.). I elaborate these basic principles because I believe the readiness to respond adequately and creatively to a dilemma posed lies at the heart of living with one's fate adaptively throughout life and is the basis of acquiring a heuristic approach, as described above. The capacity to turn towards a traumatic truth or evidence of a singular or collective wound takes courage and embraces the art of spiritual and/ or mindfulness practices. See also K. B. Tauvon's application of depth psychology in psychodramatic work in "Psychodrama and Group-Analytic Psychotherapy" (2005).
6 In Jungian psychology, the trickster figure can be seen as a disruptor of the order of things where one is exposed to the shadow (what is unconscious) part of one's psyche or that of a collective. If unheeded, the trajectory of individuation will be

hampered, slowed, deadened. We will see how Lucas's psychodrama had such an effect by bringing the reality of impending death out into the center of the room and our awareness.

7 The poem by Mawlana Jalal-al-al Din Rumi is entitled "There is some kiss we want with our whole lives": There is some kiss we want with our whole lives, the touch of spirit on the body ... At night I open the window and ask the moon to come and press its face against mine and breathe into me. Close the language-door and open the love-window. The moon won't use the door, only the window (Rumi, 2021).

8 Lucas's request that I be with him during his death is an example of a dual role. Graham engages with this topic in Chapter 3, and I address the topic further in my relationship with Greg Fowler in the final section of this chapter.

9 A month following this drama, I gifted Lucas a bar of French triple-milled soap. He roared with laughter and appreciation because I was keeping his death request in mind. Lucas's actual dying process was not exactly as he had or could foresee, although the spirit of his wishes was honored.

10 I have in various forms used this vignette for different purposes (Brooks, 2018, 2022). In this book, my purpose is to clinically illustrate how a transformative collective response (what I have elsewhere referred to as trans-subjective) may lead to a group's individuation over time. My interpretation of this scene engaged a loose reading of Jacques Lacan's 1945 essay that I have described at length elsewhere (Lacan, 2006; Brooks, 2022).

11 I am grateful to Kim David Hall for the term *puniverse.*

12 It is impossible to name everyone who participated in Quest or Team Quest activities, including allies whose contributions bolstered the momentum of what often enough felt like a hopeless cause (AIDS pandemic) The two YouTube videos produced by Fowler (2006) and Carloss (2012) of the Rainer and Kilimanjaro climbs, respectively, not only name the climbers but also give the viewer a more poignant sense of what climbing a mountain is like for a person living with HIV/AIDS, or any of us.

13 See David France's autoethnographic and historical account of gay rights activism entitled *How to Survive a Plague: The Story of How Activists and Scientists Tamed Aids* (2016). Activism and science eventually shaped the outcome of the AIDS epidemic while society and government virtually ignored its uncontained deadly spread. See also Sarah Shulman's historical recapitulation of ACT UP New York in the early years of the plague and how crucial the movement was in changing the course of care for those living with HIV/AIDS (Shulman, 2021). Activists became their own lobbyists, drug smugglers, researchers, and media specialists (journals and newspapers) to force reform at all levels of the nation's institutions, disease-fighting agencies, and policy. Also see Perry Halkitis's account of the survival strategies of the first generation of those infected with HIV/AIDS entitled *The AIDS Generation: Stories of Survival and Resilience* (2015).

References

Attinello, P. (2023). Splintered Afterlives: AIDS, Death and Beyond. In E. Brodersen (Ed.), *Jungian Dimensions on the Mourning Process, Burial Rituals and Access to the Land of the Dead: Intimations of Immortality*, pp. 71–83. New York and London: Routledge.

Boulé, M. (1999, August 9). A Sporting Chance for HIV Patients? You Betcha. *The Oregonian.*

Boulé, M. (1999, August 15). From the Deathbed to Summit. *The Oregonian.*

Brooks, R. M. (2018). Self as Political Possibility: Subversive Neighbor Love and Transcendental Agency amidst Collective Blindness. *International Journal of Jungian Studies*, 10(1), 48–75.

Brooks, R. M. (2022). *Catastrophe, Psychoanalysis and Social Change*. New York: Routledge.

Carloss, C. (2012, June 7). *Climb for Life*. Eds. G. Fowler and C. Carloss. [Video]. YouTube: https://youtu.be/Q1jPkj32zHA. Accessed May 22, 2018.

Christakis, N. (2019). *Blueprint: The Evolutionary Origins of a Good Society*. New York: Little, Brown Spark.

Dudley, S. (1999, March 5). No Mountain High Enough: Team Quest Offers Challenges and Community to Combat Illness and Despair. *The Oregonian*.

Dudley, S. (1999, August 9). Adventurous Team Quest Reaches Beyond Disabilities. *The Oregonian*.

France, D. (2016). *How to Survive a Plague: The Story of How Activists and Scientists Tamed AIDS*. New York: Alfred A. Knopf.

Fowler, G. (1999). Perspectives from the Top. *Oregon and S.W. Washington HIV Positive Letter*.

Fowler, G. (2006, March 13). Mount Rainier Climb with Project Quest. Videographer, Christopher Carloss [Video]. YouTube. https://youtu.be/HGptSPJuyhI. Accessed September 12, 2018.

Goodwyn, E. (2015). The End of All Tears: A Dynamic Interdisciplinary Analysis of Mourning and Complicated Grief with Suggested Applications for Clinicians. *Journal of Spirituality in Mental Health*, 17(4), 239–266.

Halkitis, P. (2015). *The AIDS Generation: Stories of Survival and Resilience*. New York: Cambridge University Press.

Kristeva, J. (1987). *Woman Alterity* (M. C. Taylor, Ed.). Chicago, IL and London: University of Chicago Press.

Lacan, J. (2006). *Ecrits*. Translated by Bruce Fink. New York and London: W. W. Norton.

Martín-Baró, I. (1994). *Writings for a Liberation Psychology*. Cambridge, MA: Harvard University Press.

McGonigal, K. (2015). *The Upside of Stress: Why Stress Is Good for You and How to Get Good at It*. New York: Avery.

Moreno, J. L. (1955). Sociometry and the Science of Man. *Sociometry*, 18(4), 105–118.

Moreno, J. L. (1953). *Who Shall Survive?* New York: Beacon House.

Moreno, J. L. (1946). *Psychodrama*. Vol. 1. New York: Beacon Hill.

Rumi, M. (2021, April 1). Some Kiss We Want. www.best-poems.net/rumi/some_kiss_we_want.html. Accessed October 12, 2019.

Schulman, S. (2021). *Let the Record Show: A Political History of ACT UP New York, 1987–1993*. New York: Farrar, Straus and Giroux.

Tauvon, K. B. (2005). Psychodrama and Group-Analytic Psychotherapy. In M. Karp, P. Holmes, & K. B. Tauvon (Eds.), *Handbook of Psychodrama*, pp. 277–296. London and New York: Routledge.

Ulon, S. & Brooks, R. M. (2018). Collective Shadows on the Sociodrama Stage. *International Journal of Jungian Studies*, 10(3), 221–236.

Williams, A. (1991). *Forbidden Agendas: Strategic Action in Groups*. London and New York: Tavistock/Routledge.

Part III

Re-visioning the Nonprofit Clinic, Public Program Administration, and Depth Psychology in Mental Health Today

Chapter 7

Re-visioning the Nonprofit Clinic

Lusijah Marx

How Project Quest Moved Forward

Over the last 35 years, the world has undergone profound transformations, and the Quest Center for Integrative Health in Oregon is no exception. Since its founding during the AIDS crisis in 1989, Project Quest has weathered significant changes in its mission, structure, and funding sources while striving to serve its community with empowerment, healing, and social justice at its core.

After its founding, as the Quest community grew, the need for a stronger infrastructure became apparent. To expand its impact and address the pressing mental health and addiction issues in the HIV-positive community, the organization transitioned to a nonprofit structure in 1989. Becoming a 501(c)3 nonprofit organization allowed Quest to access more funding sources, including government support, and to offer donors tax deductions for their contributions.

While this shift provided financial stability, it also introduced new challenges, such as the need to compete for grants and comply with funding requirements. It was always important to me that we remain a "center" or "community-based program." I never wanted Quest to become what I call an "agency." In my work experience, I've found that agencies tend to take away the agency from the people. When that happens, access is limited in various ways. There are many policies and procedures instated to ensure the safety, boundaries, and functioning of everyone. Pleasing funders can define what happens more than the needs of the people, and rules and paperwork shut down spontaneity and creativity. As a hierarchy forms, decisions are often made by just a few people, based on how well they can navigate power structures.

We were fortunate to have Graham, who was one of the first therapists at Quest, to help us figure out how to use our nonprofit status to get funds so our community could thrive and people could get paid to work there. Finally, we could hire people, rent space, and have basic office equipment while doing all the tracking that government funding required. It also allowed us to apply for Ryan White HIV/AIDS federal funding, which began in 1991. Our community members took on most of the needed functions, such as answering phones, setting up

DOI: 10.4324/9781003386339-11

services for people, arranging help for those in need, and planning memorials for those who died. Brian Bounous, our first official board chair, was answering phones and engaged with others up until three days before he died. Jack Cox, a loving father figure for many who were infected, handled our finances and bookkeeping and made sure we stayed within our budget. Lucas Harris, co-founder, helped build the community with his vibrant spirit and outreach to those in need. It was a very challenging time but filled with purpose and love.

Growing Pains

As we gained more ease as an organization in paying the rent and developing a paid staff, we continually grieved losses. Most of our time was spent holding our community together by helping those who were sick and supporting each other to stay as healthy and connected to self and others as possible.

With the advent of antiretrovirals in the mid-1990s, Quest changed. Our focus had always been on "living life fully," which included death as a part of life. The combination of antiretrovirals, which were improving as they developed, changed our focus too. Many of our community members needed therapy that focused on the trauma of the pandemic and continued treatment for pain, addiction issues, grief, and living with a chronic illness. The emphasis shifted to empowering a community now dealing with the perspective of living a longer life.

When highly active antiretroviral therapy (HAART) became available in 1996, it greatly lengthened the lifespan of people with AIDS, though it required taking many pills every day and the side effects and multiple doses made the treatment difficult. In 1997, the FDA approved Combivir, a pill that was easier to take. There was so much loss, stigma, and devastation that community continued to be essential, and we collaborated with more programs as we needed to work together. While the new medications saved lives, they also often brought side effects that were unsightly and caused various health issues, like kidney stones, gastrointestinal discomfort, and neuropathies. Integrated care with acupuncture, massage, and naturopathic treatments continued to be an important part of Quest.

After becoming a nonprofit, government funding played a pivotal role in sustaining the organization, which in turn mandated adherence to regulations and accountability requirements. Initially, our board of directors came from the HIV community, and most of them supported Quest daily as volunteers. Now there was a growing need for a board of directors with diverse skills, such as accounting and legal knowledge, and that led to changes in the organizational structure. Our new board had a lawyer, an accountant, and a person who had fundraising experience. The board, in conjunction with the Quest staff, changed our mission from being focused on HIV to include all people with chronic illness and people seeking wellness-based healthcare.

Project Quest initially had a structure of contract workers, but with our new board, those of us working at Quest became employees. Our board helped us develop a structure with more in-house administration, bringing both more stability to the work and more demands. Project Quest was renamed the Quest Center for Integrative Health in 2005. We were no longer a "project," having established ourselves as part of the network of community-based programs serving the LGBTQ+ community in Portland, Oregon. Despite our growth and success though, we faced obstacles in maintaining our original sense of community and the freedom to explore innovative treatments.

Our board of directors saw the need for stronger fiscal management and made the decision to hire an executive director. David Eisen had been actively involved on the HIV Planning Council that helped govern how Ryan White money was spent, and we had turned to him years before when we could not find a place we could afford to rent. As Quest was beginning, we had been in the basement of the large community acupuncture program treating addiction that he directed in downtown Portland. He knew our struggles, and our mission and values resonated with him. David became our executive director in 2005, bringing strong leadership and his vision of what Quest could be.

Quest developed an addiction program, Finding and Sustaining Recovery (FSR), and hired the needed staff for treatment, managing finances and grants, and compiling reports to the county required for our funding. Additional staffers joined the HIV program, including a coordinator for Women of Wisdom (WOW) and several peer mentors. Quest also started a program for people with chronic pain who had become addicted to opiates called Wellness, Integrity, Sustaining Health (WISH).

From 2005 on, we continued to grow and provide services to marginalized people in general, with a focus on the LGBTQ+ community. David was a strong believer in "peer support," which was included in each program, and which has always brought a greater "mutual aid" feeling to the work at Quest than if we had just had "professionals." He believed in the value of our psychodrama retreats and knew how important such experiential community activities were to me, even though any activity that is not on the premises of one's organization has more liability. David even supported retreats we had in Montana, where we were able to stay in a place near Glacier National Park without paying rent.

On these adventures, we carpooled together, did yoga in a meadow, swam in the lakes, taught authentic communication, and helped people build trust in living. Creating these experiences together, our community developed needed skills—including how to have fun and feel connection and joy. Despite the challenges posed by a capitalist-based funding system, Quest persevered in serving disenfranchised communities, embracing the spirit of mutual aid that had shaped its early years.

Values, Compromises, and Deep Questions

As the Quest Center grew, we increasingly relied on government funds to expand our services. This growth allowed us to reach more people, but it also came at a cost. Over time, I became aware of how the "system" functions to preserve the wealth and power of the rich, and how I, too, inadvertently participated in this system.

The rich maintain a buffer zone that prevents those at the bottom of the economic ladder from organizing, ensuring that those with status and money remain in control. This buffer zone provides limited support to the poor, keeping hope alive while controlling those who seek systemic change. Many nonprofits in the U.S. are rooted in colonization and oppression, with those higher up in the hierarchy earning more and holding the control. Social justice focused community organizations often compromise their missions to secure funding, including Quest.

As much as I value social justice, even now I participate in an oppressive system as I compromise my integrity by "playing the game" I need to play in order to receive payment and to create the revenue to pay Quest's expenses, such as salaries, benefits, and rent. For someone to receive services at Quest, they must go through the dreaded "intake process." As a psychotherapist, it falls on me to provide a medical diagnosis as per the Diagnostic Statistical Manual (DSM V), since the insurance requirements, whether commercial, Medicaid, or Medicare, demand a medical diagnosis for reimbursement.

Quest relies on Medicaid, and the mental health assessment must be approved by a medical professional, adding more bureaucracy and cost to the process. Although I often don't believe my clients have a "medical disorder"—many of them are going through difficult life events, such as coping with a terminal illness—I give them one (for example, F41.1 Generalized Anxiety Disorder) to ensure they can access insurance-funded services, which also generate income for the organization. This compromises my integrity, and I feel conflicted about participating in a system that I believe perpetuates systemic oppression. A lot of the people I see are grappling with intense suffering brought on by losses or traumas they've experienced, and do not simply fit into a medical diagnosis.

Though we strive to maintain our social justice values, Quest must navigate a capitalistic/colonial system where many people remain ineligible for services. Since the insurance system requires medical diagnoses for reimbursement, this leads to a disconnection between the actual needs of individuals and the imposed labels. At the same time, the bureaucratic requirements for funding lead to staff burnout and reduced time for meaningful interactions. Sessions are cut short as paperwork takes precedence, and the depth of listening and care is diminished. Even if a person is referred to another agency, they might wait six months or more for an appointment.

One of my longtime clients, James (his name is changed to protect his privacy) stands as a poignant example. I first met him in the 1980s when he was just 17 and diagnosed with AIDS. James is intelligent, but his impoverished family couldn't provide the education he desired, and living in rural Oregon he was stigmatized. He hitchhiked to Los Angeles, acquiring HIV along the way, at a time when AIDS was a death sentence. Later he lived with the loss of his closest friends dying and his own struggles to survive. His health has deteriorated over time as he's faced illnesses that drain his energy and prevent him from being able to maintain a job. He spirals down, experiencing pain and fatigue while living without a home. James applied for disability but was denied, and his appeal remains pending many months later. He struggles to generate income and find a stable place to live, caught in the web of our flawed system.

My Changing Role

When I co-founded Quest with Lucas Harris, as a nonprofit our vision was to empower marginalized individuals and create a strong community for our members. But as Quest grew, I felt a loss of agency for the people seeking services, and the sense of community that once thrived began to fade. Meanwhile, I found myself having to circumvent the system to help those in need, even seeing some people without charge because they couldn't access specialized treatment within Quest. For example, it was a battle to set up a supportive art group with talented volunteers, a gifted art therapist, and an art professor. The art therapist who was initially referred for support during the pandemic was unable to facilitate the group due to a rule stating she couldn't participate as a therapy client. I had to find a workaround so she could continue as a facilitator.

My leadership role also changed over time. In 2007, I was given the title of "Clinical Director," but it felt more like a token gesture than a meaningful role. Decisions and clinical focus were now primarily determined by the leadership team, leaving me with less influence on the direction of Quest. My creative ideas were met with resistance, and I needed approval from those in charge to proceed with any new initiatives.

One such instance occurred when I agreed to oversee an individual who was working towards a master's degree in mental health and needed supervised experience. I had completed intensive training in Internal Family Systems (IFS) and they wanted to be in a setting where they could use this therapeutic approach. They were a very skilled nonbinary gay trainer in IFS and were expanding their coaching role to become a mental health therapist. We planned to work together, with them using IFS, and my guiding them in the mental health perspective and diagnosis required for insurance reimbursement. This non-standard approach was met with pushback though, since it did not fit the structure in the mental health program for people in training. With my plan rejected, I felt my value diminish.

In 2005, I supervised a trainee, who attended retreats and became very engaged with our community as part of her mental health training. She had worked as a lawyer before deciding to become a therapist, and in 2006, after her year with Quest, was offered a job in the court system related to mental health because of her skills and passion in this area. She felt she could contribute the most to the welfare of the community by continuing as a lawyer, so we agreed that when she was ready to continue her vision of becoming a mental health therapist, I would supervise her for licensure. Her belief system and approach had resonated with me and I really enjoyed our work together. She contacted me in 2022, as she had been working for a year for an agency providing support for lawyers. She felt ready to move towards licensure. When I wanted to supervise her towards licensure as a professional counselor (LPC), I was told I could not supervise her at Quest as there was no place for her, while other interns continued to come on board. I advocated for her, since I knew how talented she was and that she was committed to mutual aid. The situation was very disappointing and I felt my needs were dismissed.

Soon afterwards, she and I began to form an LLC organization so she could get her supervised hours. I needed to have someone who resonated deeply with my values and more freedom to follow my inner guidance and do innovative work. It was clear that I did not have the power at Quest to implement approaches that were important to me. I began to look for other people to join us and begin a new organization where I would have the opportunity to do the work I felt inspired to do.

Considering my relationship with Quest, I remembered having been told by a mentor that once founders realize they are in a lesser role and no longer have power or influence, they must decide for themselves a role they can live with or establish a "quitting time," or it will be decided for them. The manner in which founders tackle their leadership transition is important since, unfortunately, their emotional strengths can become a liability as the organization moves into the colonial model. Things change as the organizational structure, with its policies and procedures, becomes stronger, while spontaneity and community input and engagement become less. There is not the freedom to respond in the moment, to brainstorm and welcome every idea. Even with my love for Quest, I knew that I would need to form another smaller organization where I could feel supported in developing mutual aid and innovative treatments for all people seeking holistic healthcare.

Revival of Mutual Aid

During the COVID-19 pandemic, the isolation took a toll on our clients' mental health, prompting us to explore ways to re-engage them. Wendy Neal, a Quest physician and skilled psychodramatist, and I decided to introduce the concept of "mutual aid" to build a post-pandemic community. We realized that many of the people we served were dealing with depression or social anxiety, and had experienced a number of traumas with little support. Believing in themselves and having the confidence and trust to be included and offer something valuable was a significant challenge for them. When I presented the idea to the leadership group, they didn't offer help in implementing it, but fortunately they did not disapprove of the plan and the project moved forward.

Wendy and I aimed to develop a mutual aid–based community at Quest to help each individual feel more connected and self-reliant rather than to find themselves constantly seeking answers from providers. Active engagement was crucial in addressing depression, and supporting fellow members of a community could help people break free from isolation, leading to a more enriched and interconnected life. By nurturing a sense of belonging and empowering individuals to rely on one another, we hoped to create a more vibrant environment for everyone at Quest. We launched our community-building project, called "Mutual Aid," to involve collaborative groups forming an egalitarian system of caring and addressing issues collectively.

The goal was to create small groups that would meet weekly, allowing people to get to know each other and foster trust and support. I initially invited individuals by email, explaining the concept and its purpose, sharing that the aim of mutual aid groups is to build community in an empowered way, modeled after the group that formed around Martin Luther King Jr., which was called "Beloved Community." Members of a mutual aid community get to know each other to cooperate in serving the needs of other community members, helping them to rely less on bureaucratic systems. I invited people to join Wendy and me in addressing the capitalist/colonial system that is slow to respond to people's needs and limited in what it offers. I described how Quest began as a mutual aid community with members building the trust it takes to help each other and address issues collectively, and also talked about the research on how human connections and helping each other increases a sense of well-being for those who participate. Many who joined said they looked forward to being an agent of change and developing more egalitarian models.

The model I initially designed proved too rigid, and we faced challenges in forming groups that were inclusive and sustainable. Some individuals struggled with the commitment, while others felt left out or unable to connect due to different needs and challenges. As we went through a six-month exploration of mutual aid, a community started to emerge despite some setbacks. We learned the importance of patience, flexibility, and commitment in community building. The backbone of the community was forming, with some participants taking on leadership roles and organizing events such as walks or picnic lunches in the park. A community member emerged as a leader, suggesting a creative solution to include everyone, breaking away from the structure of separate groups. Her leadership and creative solutions highlighted the importance of community members actively contributing to the process. As a therapist, I saw the potential for teaching relationship skills and providing support as the community continued to evolve.

During our first mutual aid gathering, we conducted various experiential exercises to help people get to know each other better and talk about commonalities and differences. We started with guided imagery followed by exploring a shared vision. Next was a "step-in circle" where participants could ask the question, "Who, like me, is … " followed by "living with HIV?" or "in recovery?" or "an artist or musician?" or "a person who loves outdoor activities?" During four hours of group exercises and paired conversations, our goal was for people to get to know each other and to form small support groups that would meet independently for two months before the next workshop. We made suggestions and gave examples as to how they might structure their meetings to include everyone, enjoy the time, and deepen a sense of trust.

Several small mutual aid groups emerged, and each group had its unique dynamics. The "Crusty Pearls" group, consisting of four women who had social skills and knew how to advocate for what they wanted, thrived and enjoyed regular in-person meetings, organizing potlucks and walks. On the other hand, a group of individuals who didn't have these same advantages struggled to establish ground rules, such as a consistent time for groups to begin and end, and how to share in creating the structure of the group, and eventually dissolved. Another group of five, sharing complex health issues, found it challenging to commit to the mutual aid model. Some dropped out, while others joined functioning small groups.

We continued to meet as a larger group every two months, focusing on helping small groups develop skills and forming new groups. One member from the "Crusty Pearls" group shared how the mutual aid experience had been transformative for her, breaking her out of a pattern of limiting personal sharing, learned from her culture and family. She expressed feeling a sense of belonging and greater contentment developing from being part of the group.

As we progressed to our fourth workshop, we had new participants joining the process. We engaged in role plays, dyads, and experiential group work to foster deeper connections and understanding. The process of selecting support groups, however, presented challenges as people had varying needs and wishes. Struggles with scheduling and personal preferences often determined group dynamics.

One participant, who had experienced a traumatic brain injury and faced isolation, expressed the need for a weekly group to stay on track, but most others preferred biweekly meetings, causing her to feel frustrated and left out. The group faced a deadlock until another woman, a group member and community dinner volunteer, suggested that people could be part of more than one group, fostering greater flexibility and inclusion. As the facilitator, I learned valuable lessons about the importance of being flexible and patient in community building, and recognized that forming inclusive, sustainable groups takes time and commitment. Although some participants dropped out, it was not a failure but a natural part of the process. The collective was strengthening, and more activities and engagement were anticipated in the future. While we faced challenges, the seeds of a more natural, deeply felt community had been sown.

A New Horizon: Redwood Collaborative

Despite my admiration for Quest and the difference it makes in people's lives, I knew that my needs and aspirations would be better met in a smaller organization where I could freely engage in the creative work I longed to do. By 2022, as I mentioned, I was in the process of forming a different entity. I contacted a social worker colleague who left Quest a few years ago, due partly to the number of clients a therapist was required to see, as well as her need for more autonomy. We had trained together with Internal Family Systems in-person training and developed appreciation and trust in each other.

Yearning for a place where community, creativity, and mutual aid thrived, my colleagues and I envisioned the Redwood Collaborative, where we could continue making a meaningful impact on people's lives. My desire for a new, more flexible environment especially began to grow after a transformative experience two years ago. A woman who was seeing me for therapy, who had a terminal cancer diagnosis, invited me to attend a presentation by a New York University team on the use of psilocybin for end-of-life anxiety. Witnessing the profound benefits of psychedelic-assisted therapy for these individuals ignited my spirit. As I read studies and watched videos, I knew this was an area that I would pursue so I could facilitate healing through non-ordinary consciousness experiences.

I became aware that my fixed mindset, with a bias against psychedelics, had limited me. As a person who has been engaged in daily meditation, I had never used psychedelics or cannabis. I had images from the 1970s of people taking psychedelics and the message at the time of the "flower people" who checked out from society. Somehow, I had carried a negative feeling about hallucinogens in general and would never have imagined that I would personally have a psychedelic experience, let alone become a facilitator. But that shifted as I listened to Gabor Maté, Bessel van der Kolk, and Dick Schwartz, all persons who have such in-depth experience in dealing with trauma, agree that psychedelics offered an effective way of addressing PTSD, addictions, anxiety, and depression.

More and more, my inner guidance was letting me know that I should become a psychedelic facilitator. Oregon had passed Measure 109 in 2020, which was opening the door to the legal use of psilocybin in our state. While my guidance felt clear, I had still never experienced taking a psychedelic. I knew if I was going to work with psilocybin, it would be necessary for me to have a journey with this medicine.

My personal psilocybin experience began with a retreat in Jalisco, Mexico, which was facilitated by a shaman trained in Ecuador and her helpers. On my first retreat, as I began to feel my usual state of consciousness disappear, I experienced a special guide who was playing a flute and drawing me into a spacious place. As time progressed, I felt like dancing and singing, with my arms moving a lot to the music, and I felt the souls of many of the people I knew who had died of AIDS. I was with my beloved Lucas, along with Roger, Micah, and Luke. Brian and Jack joined us. With all of them, I could see their faces as they were when I knew them. I did not feel sadness but a part of all things. They encouraged me to be a guide and I knew it was a calling for me.

I returned to Portland, where I immersed myself in the psychedelic community and enrolled in both the California Institute of Integral Studies (CIIS) psychedelic training program and a training program in Oregon for people becoming facilitators called Inner Trek. I attended two other psilocybin retreats over the year in Morelos for guidance, to experience personal healing, and to learn skills. These experiences brought me clarity and to a beautiful, strong, spiritual state. My third trip to Mexico was to learn about psilocybin use from Indigenous women, respecting the roots of this medicine. I was aware of the dangers of psychedelics becoming co-opted by corporate greed and wanted to honor Indigenous knowledge in my education and practice. My experience, especially with a Mazateca woman from Oaxaca, was profound and empowered me to proceed.

The psychedelic training programs I attended emphasized the importance of the highest level of ethics and integrity, and for each person becoming a psychedelic guide to commit to making psychedelics available to all people, not just people with money. There was also a focus on Indigenous knowledge and sacred plants, diversity, equity and inclusion, gender and queer issues, social justice, and Indigenous reciprocity. Through my psychedelic training and experiences at CIIS and Inner Trek, I have gained understanding and a deep willingness to harness my half-century of experience to develop new healing models that emphasize community.

In making that shift I felt a growing need to share visions and dreams, as in the early days of Quest. Part of my wish in developing the organization with my colleagues is to have the freedom to choose who I work with without the constraints I've faced for years. Collaborating with a small group of like-minded people, who share a passion for innovative work and value the power of psychedelics and of collective healing, we'll work to create an environment where those who come for services can support one another, fostering a sense of belonging, purpose, and personal agency.

As a woman of 79, I recognize the importance of addressing the needs of older individuals who may internalize feelings of being overlooked or irrelevant. I believe my years of rich experience and personal growth contribute to a unique perspective that can benefit older people seeking connection and fulfillment. I envision creating a community where all individuals, including older adults, feel valued, connected, and purposeful. Supporting elders in channeling our collective wisdom for much-needed change is a vision I hold dear. With that focus, I hope to establish a community where the clinical use of psilocybin, MDMA, and other entheogens can address trauma and depression, as well as strengthen connected authentic relationships and creativity, moving beyond the boundaries of traditional therapeutic paradigms.

My goal is to explore how a mutual aid culture can be integrated into the use of entheogens in my new work setting. Focusing on addressing collective trauma, physical illness, addictions, depression, anxiety, and end-of-life concerns, my aim is to build trust, connections, and intuition within a community format. I plan to organize retreats with comprehensive preparation, offering multiple psychedelic experiences with ample support and ongoing integration over several months.

While I pursue my passion for psychedelic work, I also intend to continue cultivating the mutual aid community at Quest, where I will remain part time. I am deeply grateful for all that I have learned throughout my journey, and am committed to moving away from colonial systems and the medical model as much as possible. My aspiration is to create a more compassionate, just, and empowering world through the integration of a forward-looking approach. More recently, I was introduced to another potential avenue for psychedelic-assisted therapy—ketamine. Previously unfamiliar with ketamine and its therapeutic potential, I delved into the research and found compelling evidence for its effectiveness, and my personal experience in training for ketamine-assisted therapy (KAP) was powerful and useful.

Having begun a new chapter in my own life, I firmly believe that psychedelic-assisted therapy can open the way to creativity, connection, and profound change, and that older adults are the group I most want to support. At the Redwood Collaborative that dissolved and emerged as a nonprofit called Radiance Integrative Health and Wellness, I hope to create an affirming community with a focus on older individuals, as we all grow together. Through mutual aid and collective support, I intend to foster an environment where each person can thrive, letting go of limiting beliefs and embracing their innate wisdom and potential. By aligning with one's true self, we can all lead fuller lives and engage in purposeful endeavors that contribute positively to society. I believe in the transformative power of community, where members inspire and uplift each other, forging life-changing connections that encourage personal growth as well as deeper, more meaningful relationships with others. My vision for Radiance Integrative Health and Wellness is to be a beacon of hope and healing, where people of all ages, and especially those who are older, can find purpose, joy, and fulfillment through shared experiences and collaborative efforts.

Chapter 8

Community Empowerment in Public Program Administration

Graham Harriman

In this chapter, I reflect on how my earlier experiences as an AIDS therapist and activist for three decades inform my contemporary critique of HIV public health and mental health program administration today. I underscore the need to adopt mutual aid cultures at all levels of public policy development, from the grassroots up, so that resources are equitably shared and the project design is collectively problem solved. I propose a broadened definition of care that considers how intersectional determinants of health (poverty, income, race, class, neighborhood, education, etc.) are fundamental in designing policy and procedures for the treatment and prevention of HIV. Additionally, I reflect on my participation in the culture of privilege and open my heart and mind to a variety of experiences that challenge my lack of awareness about white supremacy and contribute to subsequent life changes.

From Quest to NYC Department of Health and Mental Hygiene and the "Race to Justice"

I was a psychotherapist working with individuals and groups with Project Quest until 2002, when I became interested in developing equitable models of care at the policy level. My initial shift to community mental health focused on identifying and engaging people in need of behavioral health services and HIV care through bilingual and bicultural mental health peer navigators and psychotherapists. A few years later, I transitioned within the Multnomah County Health Department (MCHD) to plan and administer Ryan White funding, a federal resource for U.S. cities addressing the needs of low-income people with HIV (PWH). This was a unique aspect of this federal funding, thanks to HIV advocacy involved in legislation development. Ryan White Part A Programs are required to have an appointed community planning body, comprised of at least 33% of PWH. The committee sets allocations, priorities, and guidance for HIV care and support services (Community HIV/AIDS Training and Technical Assistance, 2018, p. 3). After several years at MCHD, I also became the co-chair of the Diversity and Quality team, and then led the HCV, HIV, STI program.

DOI: 10.4324/9781003386339-12

I moved to New York from Portland, Oregon, in 2010 seeking new challenges to address equity on a larger and more complex scale. In Portland, I noticed that white people could work on issues of inclusion but had fewer opportunities to actually address their own biases because they were insulated from communities of color, as I was. My move to New York allowed me to rigorously interrogate my biases as a middle-class, white, gay man, with HIV. My participation in a bureaucracy has perpetuated inequitable access to resources, health, education, and quality of life even if the program's purpose is creating equitable access to care and improved health. I've made it my personal and professional work to identify the structures that I have participated in with the health department that contribute to inequitable access to resources, growth, and health. The NYC Department of Health's "Race to Justice Initiative" informs and steers that transformation.

Following my move to NYC in 2010, I joined the NYC Department of Health and Mental Hygiene (DOHMH) in the HIV Care and Treatment Program, which is responsible for the Ryan White Part A funding for NYC and the TriCounty area (Rockland, Putnam, and Westchester counties). Moving from a small jurisdiction to a larger one required an even stronger and multifaceted community planning effort. This is the largest jurisdiction with what is arguably the most diverse population in the United States, with entrenched issues of racism, sexism, poverty, and classism.

After several years at DOHMH, in 2014, NYC Mayor Bill Deblasio appointed Mary Basset, MD, MPH (Wortsman, 2015) as the Commissioner of Health for DOHMH. Dr. Basset became responsible for leading the department charged with the health of the largest and most diverse city in the U.S. NYC has over 8.5 million people, with a minority identifying as white non-Hispanic (31.9%), 28.9% as Latino, 23.4% as Black, and 14.2% as Asian/Asian American, and 37% of the residents born outside of the United States (NYC Mayor's Office for Economic Opportunity, 2020; U.S. Census Bureau, 2021). Through Dr. Bassett's leadership, public health shifted to center community engagement while explicitly addressing racism, poverty, and other social determinants of health. Dr. Bassett formed an initiative called *Race to Justice* with the following statement framing this work. Bassett stated:

> Every New Yorker deserves to achieve their full health potential. However, not everyone has fair access to the factors that contribute to good health, such as healthy foods, safe places to live and play, and a wage that allows them to live with dignity.
>
> This is unjust. To address this, the Race to Justice had three strategies:

- Study how racism has affected our past work and create new policies to lessen that impact.

- Educate and train staff on how racism and other systems of oppression can shape health.
- Collaborate with local communities to counter injustices.

(NYC Health, 2016a)

Regarding the contradictions that are already in place to make such a change, Wortsman stated: "One of the central aspects of public health is to gather data, and use it to make decisions to improve health. However, in the area of race, the dominant culture can often disregard data, in its effort to maintain the status quo, consciously and subconsciously" (Wortsman, 2015).

On several occasions, data on health inequities was presented and not accepted by white colleagues and, oftentimes, by me. Living in privilege as a white person often means that I have denied the data to maintain my comfort versus grappling with the reality of living in a racist culture. White colleagues, I noted, at DOHMH would often respond with disbelief about the data, expressing concerns about the research methodology or type of analysis conducted. For example, I specifically recall a staff survey which delineated the differing experiences of racism by Black, Latino, Asian, and white staff that was discounted by white staff. The rejection was founded on disbelief, even though the analysis had been reviewed by numerous public health professionals and was conducted by a Ph.D.-level epidemiologist.

Regardless, the data is clear. The wealth gap alone between Black and white Americans has been persistent and extreme. It represents, scholars say, the accumulated effects of four centuries of institutional and systemic racism and bears a major responsibility for disparities in income, health, education, and opportunity that continue to this day. For instance, the net wealth of a typical Black family in America is around one-tenth that of a white family. A 2018 analysis of U.S. incomes and wealth by economists Moritz Kuhn, Moritz Schularick, and Ulrike Steins, published by the Federal Reserve Bank of Minneapolis, concluded: "The historical data also reveal that no progress has been made in reducing income and wealth inequalities between Black and white households over the past 70 years" (Mineo, 2021, p. 1). With the most recent pandemic, it is more difficult for our society to be in denial about the effects of racism. In New York State during the COVID-19 surge, Black residents were more than four times more likely than white people to be hospitalized, and more than twice as likely to die. Latino residents were nearly four times more likely to be hospitalized and 70% more likely to die (COVID Tracking Project, 2021).

Decades earlier, PWH *paid for* a homophobic, racist, sexist, transphobic, and class-based society, with *our bodies*. It was a stark reality that could not be ignored within the Quest and HIV community, but was ignored by those in institutions of power. Having our lives at stake created an urgency to demand what we needed, leading to the formulation of the Denver Principles. The Principles were developed in 1983 and cogently began with this statement:

> We condemn attempts to label us as "victims," a term which implies defeat, and we are only occasionally "patients," a term which implies passivity, helplessness, and dependence upon the care of others. We are "People With AIDS."
>
> (The Denver Principles, 1983)

These principles became foundational for HIV activist work and mobilized change in the culture of healthcare, reorienting community authority over the use of funding for the needs of PWH. I believe these principles still need to guide us in public health, healthcare, and mental health HIV advocacy today.

In the early decades of AIDS, gay, white men were predominantly visible, demanding their right to treatment and to make decisions about their own sexual and physical health, in response to an ignorant government guided by homophobia (and racism and sexism). Systems of grassroots efforts were created through mass community-based volunteer efforts. Quest was a part of that effort. Survival was based on a mixture of hope, luck, and determination. We took care of each other as we struggled to survive while helping each other through diagnosis, death, and grieving.

Without any treatment available, the death rate was fairly equal among PWH, but shifted with the introduction of more effective medications. Consequently, issues regarding access to care were unmasked. White PWH fared better with post-treatment availability (Braunstein et al., 2022). It is this privilege—access to care and the social determinants that affect access to care—that must be addressed in the latest efforts to "End the HIV Epidemic" (HIV.Gov, 2023). Addressing these inequities will require each of us collectively engaging with structural racism, sexism, homophobia, and transphobia, as well as biases regarding immigration, poverty, and geography (Bowleg et al., 2022).

The current National HIV/AIDS Plan made the following observations:

> … unavailability of access to HIV healthcare and testing in combination. Additionally cultural HIV/AIDS stigma has increased with the rates of delayed diagnosis and treatment. Homo-negativity in the African American population must be addressed even further, to stem the increasing incidence of HIV/AIDS amongst Black men who have sex with men or BMSM.
>
> (The White House, 2021, p. 48)

For decades, those of us working in HIV have understood that this epidemic is accelerated at the intersection of racism, homophobia, transphobia, sexism, immigration status, and poverty. This is evident in over 30 years of data illustrating patterns of poverty by neighborhood (NYC Health, 2021, pp. 13–14), inequitable rates by race/ethnicity and gender for HIV diagnoses (NYC Health, 2021, p. 16), and HIV viral load suppression (NYC Health, 2021, p. 21). The racist, classist, and transphobic elements of our society are reflected in this data as people on the margins of society pay with their health. The systems of oppression are persistent.

We can see the increased effects of intersectional oppression when we look at multiply oppressed populations. Earlier in my time at the NYC DOHMH, I admit to not fully understanding the reasons for the high rates of HIV or the lowest rates of viral suppression among Black gay men (CDC, 2018). My eyes were opened when I read a publication (Millett et al., 2012) which clearly stated that high HIV prevalence among Black men who have sex with men (Black MSM) was not due to the number of sex partners or lack of condom use. These high rates were driven by social determinants of health, including access to care and treatment, poverty, and other aspects of cultural and institutional racism. In other words, the structural inequities for Black MSM are so prevalent that individual risk factors, though they are more likely to be mitigated by Black MSM, are unimportant in reducing risk for HIV disease. The lack of access to care and resulting higher viral load creates more opportunities for HIV, and STI, infections. This is due to the higher infectiousness of those with detectable viral load, and the much higher likelihood of Black MSM choosing Black MSM partners. Yet our racist culture continues to blame individuals for societal problems.

The Millett publication outlines the need to create lasting and sustainable change in our society by looking beyond individual behaviors to counter the forces that maintain inequality. By lifting ourselves above the valued individualism that pervades our lives here in the United States, we can begin to see societal forces more clearly in their true light. Those in positions of power need to be continually reminded to let go of their egos, share leadership, and step back, which requires consistent awareness and training on the part of those at the top in a hierarchical system. The mechanisms to maintain and consolidate power are rewarded by hierarchy with promotions, increased salaries, additional resources, and privilege, making efforts at equity in an inherently inequitable system a consistent challenge.

An important component to the Race to Justice Initiative at the NYC DOHMH has been to engage staff in education and training. Training is oriented towards identifying personal, professional, and structural barriers to addressing racism in the department's work. In 2016, the NYC Bureau of HIV enrolled about 40 staffers in lead positions, including myself, in a three-day training conducted by the People's Institute for Survival and Beyond (Undoing Racism: PISAB, n.d.). The essence of the trainings sought to begin a process of untangling the many forces which perpetuate racism, which PISAB (n.d.) defines as

… the single most critical barrier to building effective coalitions for social change. Racism has been consciously and systematically erected, and it can be undone only if people understand what it is, where it comes from, how it functions, and why it is perpetuated.

The PISAB Principles outline the work that was initiated in this session and serve as a lifelong endeavor to uncover and address racism:

> Our commitment to anti-racist organizing principles is what holds our collective work together. As the forces of racism persist, anti-racist principles keep us grounded, and focused on our collective vision. We believe that an effective, broad-based movement for social transformation must be rooted in the following Anti-Racist Organizing Principles:

> * Analyzing Power
> * Developing Leadership
> * Gatekeeping
> * Identifying and Analyzing Manifestations of Racism
> * Learning from History
> * Maintaining Accountability
> * Networking
> * Sharing Culture
> * Undoing Internalized Racial Oppression (addressing Internalized Racial Inferiority and Internalized Racial Superiority).

> (PISAB, n.d.)

My experience of the PISAB training led to a profoundly personal and professional challenge to understand my role in maintaining the societal structures of racism. How was I subconsciously sustaining racist practices and the culture of white supremacy? During the training, I struggled with my identity as a person who had dedicated his career to serving my community. I was horrified with my actions that perpetuated inequality. For example, at the time, the standards of performance to which I held my team were implicitly influenced by my biased understanding of professionalism based on white supremacy. More specifically, I valued a communication style with less emotion focused on objectivity and an academic writing style that also reflected the values of the health department. During the training, I was grappling with the career I had worked to develop over 30 years to address equity, when in fact I subconsciously was perpetuating white supremacy because of my own acculturation as a white man. I was in denial of my own privilege and my privilege's effect on my decision making. Though my experience as a gay man with AIDS gives me some perspective, I had also benefited from my liberal arts education and financial support from my family when I was ill. Family support helped me to stay partially employed without having to be on disability, and my white skin lent me a much different experience than non-white PWH.

As a result of the PISAB training, I questioned my own perspectives on how to help. For decades, as a leader, I had relied on my own experience of HIV and the administrative knowledge of healthcare systems to guide decision making.

My experience as a gay white man with HIV guided many of my decisions. Even though I have much to be proud of, I discounted the effect of stigma fueled by racism, sexism, and homophobia because I had only rarely experienced such stigma. This led me to discount the effects of provider bias, which leads to inequitable care (Suluaiman, 2020). I could also discount the larger societal bias against PWH that I experienced to some degree in my professional life. However, because I'm an educated white man, I was minimally impacted in comparison to my non-white PWH professional colleagues.

What has helped me to continually transform my thinking (which will need to continue for the rest of my life) was to deepen my understanding of the culture of white supremacy. The qualities of white supremacy, as outlined by Tema Okun (Okun, 2021), include perfectionism, a sense of urgency, defensiveness and/or denial, quantity over quality, worship of the written word, the belief in one "right" way, paternalism, either/or binary thinking, power hoarding, fear of open conflict, individualism, progress defined as more, the right to profit, objectivity, and the right to comfort. I can honestly, uncomfortably, and openly say that I have every one of these qualities and see them in my white colleagues and some of my colleagues of color in positions of power on a regular basis. I can think of many times when I reacted with defensiveness or disbelief when Black and Latino/a persons shared their experience of racism.

My leadership was influenced by my cognitive biases, my worldview, perceived threat, and a need for power. I'm not proud to write this. I can also say that the department has established laws, institutional practices, and cultural norms that get in the way of promoting equity, much of which is extremely resistant to change.

Accompanying the shift under Dr. Bassett's leadership, the NYC Department of Health and Mental Hygiene embraced community engagement, stating:

> As a local public health department, we can advance justice through critical research, policy, advocacy, program development and evaluation, and other public health practices. This work includes examining the power dynamics and structures within and among the institutions—including our own—that maintain inequities. Understanding and addressing these dynamics is critical to meaningful community engagement; they determine who we choose to engage, who is included in decision-making, and how community members' power is valued and accounted for in our work.
>
> (NYC Health, 2017)

In my position as the Director of the HIV Health and Human Services Planning Council (the Council), I had the honor of leading the Ryan White Part A Planning Council with the largest grant in the nation. This grant addressed the medical and support service needs of low-income PWH. Ryan White Planning Councils are the only legislatively mandated community-driven planning process in US public health with specific responsibilities for funding allocations, priorities, and service guidance. As mentioned earlier, per the Ryan White HIV/AIDS Program legislation, the planning body must be comprised of 33% unaligned PWH, representative of the local epidemic, and include providers, public health professionals, and others with experience and knowledge of services to support the health of PWH (Community HIV/AIDS Training and Technical Assistance, 2018). The legislation was put together with many thanks to advocates who believed in the principles of community, thereby steering the use of resources towards communities of need. On numerous occasions, local governments attempted to change the Council's authority, but with no success due to the broad support of HIV advocates. In fact, the unique nature of these Councils makes them an ideal environment to center community engagement and community voice. This can be replicated to ensure community input for all uses of government funding.

In their 30-year history, HIV Planning Councils made bold decisions that haven't been initiated by government, and at times were not supported by government, due to long-standing interests in services. The locally approved New York Council directives include:

- A Framing Directive which supports the development of a system which is active in pursuing anti-racist policies, trauma-informed care, and client-centered service provision (HIV Health and Human Services Planning Council of New York, 2021a).
- A directive to support the oral health needs of PWH (HIV Health and Human Services Planning Council of New York, 2021b).
- Development of new services to meet the needs of Transgender, Intersex, Gender Non-Binary, Non-Conforming experienced PWH (HIV Health and Human Services Planning Council of New York, 2019).
- An initiative that serves to address the needs of Aging PWH (HIV Health and Human Services Planning Council of New York, 2021c).

Building on these successes is what is needed for the health of our communities and the health of PWH.

I can recall a time in my work in the HIV Planning Council when we worked to address unequal pay for people of color in NYC. We knew that HIV care services staff were poorly compensated, with many earning less than a living wage, while community-based organizations (CBO) leadership salaries vary from $120,000–400,000 annually. Most recently, the Center for New York City Affairs published a report that highlighted the poor pay for nonprofit human service staff. The report noted that 75% of the staff were persons of color, 70% of whom are women. Many providers in the committee thought that nothing could be done about pay equity due to HR policies, labor agreements, and class titles at each agency. This became a convenient excuse for lack of action and a common response from many managers (Livingston, 2020). To address this, the committee developed a pay review that would occur at each agency to measure inequity and develop plans for improvement.

Mainstream publications such as the *Harvard Business Review* are recognizing the importance of equal pay. Livingston (2020), for example states:

> Understanding an ailment's roots is critical to choosing the best remedy. Racism can have many psychological sources—cognitive biases, personality characteristics, ideological worldviews, psychological insecurity, perceived threat, or a need for power and ego enhancement. But most racism is the result of structural factors—established laws, institutional practices, and cultural norms.
>
> (Livingston, 2020)

Establishing standards and expectations for equitable pay is an important first step in addressing inequity, regardless of the difficulty in addressing the upstream causes of inequitable compensation. Systemic inequity reform takes consistent effort, with a parallel process of evaluation to determine whether changes result in the intended outcomes. The tools we have at hand in our bureaucracies are often intended to perpetuate inequity. In the era of Black Lives Matter, complicit engagement in a racist culture has promoted inequality in wages, healthcare, housing, and quality of life, leaving many white people with an experience of shame that we choose to understand or deny. We can be complicit in our privilege. We can deny marginalized persons the ability to engage in policy decisions that affect them or support their capacity to be a part of change in our culture. We do not incorporate mutual aid approaches that mobilize community members in creative, egalitarian processes for mutual exchange and social change.

In the NYC Department of Health, we were expected to publish, conduct research, be leaders for the nation, establish relationships with hospitals, clinics, academia and, often, ignore criticism. The culture of the department is competitive, data driven, and often lacks an understanding of human experience. In the time I have been at the department I have seen proposals that characterized HIV-positive gay men as vectors of disease, efforts to contain PWH who are virally unsuppressed, and statements that blame Black gay men based on perceived promiscuity. This is contrary to Millett et al.'s (2012) publication cited earlier, as well as additional publications such as Laurencin et al. (2018) that investigated stigma and homophobia.

Early on in my time in 2011 the department released an advertisement campaign that stigmatized people with HIV called "It's Never Just HIV." The campaign insinuated that side effects from antiretrovirals and the effects of having HIV led to severe bone loss and dementia—problematic on many fronts (Gaycities, 2011). The message was a misguided effort at HIV prevention, intending to scare people to remain HIV-negative, at the cost of stigmatizing PWH. The community responded to the messaging in an uproar (Horn, 2010), but the department dug in, and reiterated its belief in scare tactics, thereby ignoring valuable feedback from the community and squelching dissent. The community argued that the ad stigmatized PWH, created barriers to effective treatment for PWH, and used data out of context for its scare tactic – without offering a solution, calls for a revision of the message were completely ignored. The ad is an example of how the values of white supremacy permeate culture, resulting in people taking a defensive stance in maintaining there is only one right way to focus on a perceived threat. This was a typical approach in the health department before Mary Bassett's leadership and much of this culture continues because it is embedded in the structure of the bureaucracy that retains a rigid hierarchy in its service requirements and arguments against providing equitable pay and in diversifying leadership. There remain continued and persistent efforts to dismantle inequity advocated for in the Race to Justice program.

It's important to note that the department *has* also shifted tremendously, in the past 14 years supporting sexual health. The department has supported innovations in biomedical prevention including NYC Health, HIV: Undetectable Equals Untransmittable (U=U) (NYC Health, 2016b), and scaled-up accessibility of pre-exposure prophylaxis (PrEP) and post-exposure prophylaxis (PEP). However, a slow-to-change bureaucracy leads to burnout among the staff and leadership who are held back from being able to implement practices that uphold equity, and it contributes to the lack of ability to accept community criticism as a means of quality improvement. Products and services are difficult to procure, staff vacancies are difficult to fill, and payment of community contractors is untimely and problematic for nonprofit organizations that have extremely high rent and overhead costs (Crowe & Rosenn, 2023). It is an incredibly challenging work environment that takes years to understand, but also takes its toll over the years as the unyielding bureaucracy leads to frustration, poor morale, and learned helplessness. We have antiquated tools in bureaucracies, job titles, and classes, and ways of assigning value and worth that assign meaning to the wrong ideals. We pay more for education, we pay more for certain types of experience for a job, and we have job classes that limit the ability to hire the right people for the job. The structures we work in are ineffective. We are in a state of transition, working to create systems of equity within systems that are inherently based on inequity; the road map is unclear, being created in real time.

I struggled internally within the department to actively promote staff for raises and ensure diversity in different positions when I led the program. I did not do a good job at supporting the Black managers and staff I hired over the years. I didn't have the tools to support them and the tools I used with others weren't relevant to their needs. At times I judged them unfairly, vacillating between not providing enough guidance or too much. It was difficult to decipher if the feedback I gave was helpful or didn't resonate, given the dynamics between a white manager and Black supervisee. I was unequipped to figuring out how to support my Black colleagues and supervisees with my white supremacy cultural toolbox. I found supporting staff to be competitive, linear, focused on quantity/ productivity and individual needs versus group culture needs. I did think of joint team projects to address inequities, and most recently I moved positions to allow increased diversity in leadership. I now realize that my place is to support change, not to lead change. I can't say I've done this gracefully or perfectly, but I've tried to remain open to feedback and open to forward motion. Learning what does and does not work while creating an equitable, open process for centering community and social justice can't be done without humility and reflection. This was our approach when I worked with the Quest community decades ago. We had to be flexible and open to the needs of community members in program development and group psychotherapy. I recognize that I haven't known and often still don't know how to advocate for my BIPOC peers and supervisees in the workplace. I've come to a place of trying to do the least harm. I attempt to step back and let others lead when possible and lead through collaboration.

My Departure, Stepping Back and Forward

As I began to prepare for my departure from the program, I noticed there were efforts to reign in control and marginalize community input. This began when a person who worked for me spoke out directly to a government representative in power, coupled with a tone that put people on the defensive. I was instructed to place the individual on disciplinary status. As a dutiful government employee, at first I complied but then realized it was the dynamics of a hierarchy keeping dissent in check. I could not, by any stretch of the imagination, be responsible for placing my supervisee in jeopardy because they were describing their experience. I encouraged the employee to comply with the HR plan so that they would not be at further risk. Consequently, the department was separated from the Council staff, 15 floors below, so that there would be less engagement and conflict. Meetings were refused between one department and another, and communication about what was happening was cut off. Furthermore, the lead person publicly stated on national calls that the other department's authority was not needed and the legislation needed to be changed. The justification for these actions was that the government understood the needs of PWH 30 years into the epidemic, and there wasn't a need for community to give input on how to spend the funding.

It became clearer and clearer to me that I needed to make a strong stand for community input. It wasn't a time to be nice and try for diplomacy, to find a middle road—there was no acceptable middle road. One night I looked for guidance in the *Pedagogy of the Oppressed* by Paulo Freire (1995). This statement resonated with me strongly:

> Solidarity with the oppressed requires that one enter into the situation of those with whom one is identifying; it is a radical posture. If what characterizes the

oppressed is their subordination to the consciousness of the master, as He-gel affirms, true solidarity with the oppressed means fighting at their side to transform the objective reality which has made them "beings for another."

(Freire, 1995, p. 12)

It was what I knew intuitively. I needed to work directly with PWH, drawing on one of Dean Spade's three key elements of mutual aid: "Mutual aid projects are participatory, solving problems for collective action rather than waiting for saviors" (Spade, 2020, p. 12). One consumer decided that it would make sense to have a separate meeting of PWH to come to a consensus on how they wanted to address the situation since they too felt marginalized, noticing the poor tone of government representation in meetings, the lack of response to consumer emails to the program director, the lack of response from lines of questioning from the Council, and a disregard for consumer input into the service system. In the last Council meeting I co-directed, I made a point of putting on record what was at risk—the very spirit of the legislation centering community input on the program.

The process of writing this book, combined with my decision to leave my position in the health department, led me to step into radicalization. I am able to dream of a place that isn't ruled by institutions or agencies and to return to where Quest (with empowerment) began: centering community. Going back to the well … and effectively responding to community. I need to revisit the roots of my personal and professional life by following what resonates with my integrity.

As I began to prepare for my departure from the health department while working on this chapter, little did I know that the very essence of what we are focusing on in this book would come front and center in my work today. I have come full circle, reflecting on how government can support community engage-ment. I've spent my career straddling the inside world of being a provider or public health director while also being a person who has lived 33 years with HIV.

In the past several years it has become apparent to me that I have been main-taining the status quo by holding a position of power. Holding onto my place in leadership as a gay white man with HIV in his mid-fifties is a trend we see in the field of HIV. Those of us who connected to the field in our twenties came to the work with a sense of purpose, passion, and commitment to our commu-nity. The disease was different in the 1980s and 1990s. Since then, the epidemi-ology has shifted, our culture has shifted, and it is past time for a new generation of activists to take the reins. HIV leadership is most effective comprised of those who directly experienced the inequities inflicted by white supremacy, in order to undo unjust practices through policy implementation and to mobilize a deeper societal transformation.

However, in stepping back I am also aware that the power dynamics of gov-ernment create their own means of marginalizing community through structur-ally racist practices embedded in the culture of hierarchical bureaucracy, which gives no guarantee that the work will change in a way that more actively centers community. I made a conscious decision to continue to support and coach those in leadership to create new systems of change in the services they oversee. I think I can be an effective ally by supporting change from behind the scenes and on an individual basis. I am returning to my roots as a psychotherapist but informed by decades of government leadership experience. I'm thankful I kept my license as a practicing counselor current all these years to be able to make this transition.

Post departure, I commit myself to ensuring PWH and the community are vocal and empowered to guide services. Through support and raising my own awareness, I can support processes and structures that allow for diverse voices and better define my role as an ally for social change and equity. By going back to community and out of the hierarchy of government, I seek to create change from an angle that I think it more appropriate for this middle-aged, white, gay, HIV-positive man. My next effort to address equity will be through a supportive role and not through the role of top-down leadership.

I'm reminded of Moreno's concept of the Godhead (Moreno, 1978, p. xix) that was crucial for centering community engagement, as echoed in Quaker-ism, Kundalini yoga, and other spiritual influences which center knowledge and guidance within, versus from above or outside. This concept can be described spiritually but it can also be described sociologically and psychologically as centering one's locus of control to create agency in one's life and connecting in community. It is this dynamic that is essential to consumer empowerment and community engagement, emphasizing what one needs and what the group needs, and taking collective action to secure that need. What this requires is a governmental system that values mutuality in relationship with the community it serves to improve mental health or healthcare systems. Power is shared, not horded. Power is distributed. Collaboration requires that those in power step back and listen to those in need, so that problems can be effectively solved. As Paulo Freire explains it, oppression by one group over another is commonplace in terms of being the "result of an unjust order that engenders violence in the op-pressors, which in turn dehumanizes the oppressed" (Freire, 1995, p. 26). What is also crucial is that both the oppressor and the oppressed are dehumanized by the relationship of exploitation permeating their collective society.

We have yet to develop tools to dismantle oppression on a personal, profes-sional, and organizational level. The health department has publicly stated that it needs to address systems of oppression internally and externally; however, the tools it employs for addressing disagreements between those in authority and staff are antiquated and built on maintaining order and respect towards those in decision-making roles—a recipe for continuing systemic racism. The system is broken. People in positions of power must better understand and reflect on our own culture of privilege and open our hearts and minds to shared leadership or, even better, following community leadership in our managerial practices and bureaucratic structures.

The acts of engaging, witnessing, and being present changed the experiences of people with AIDS (PWA) and allowed for innovative models of care to emerge that transformed how we worked with community, death, illness, and medical care. It was not just the experience of those who were challenged with HIV, but it also became the experience of those who took up the challenge of supporting PWH. I could not have made it to this day without my HIV-negative allies and support network, my partner, my doctor, my friends, and, of course, my work colleagues. The same is true for so many others, then and now. The ability to harness hope and live through the challenging time is not just the work of the individual, but the work of the community that we chose to engage with. *Quest provided that space in its organic imperfection.* We were all called to be there for each other in a process of collective empowerment and healing. My hope is that mutual aid–based approaches will be more broadly applied to public program administration and other environments, including climate change, political systems, and all other areas of life.

References

Bowleg, L., Malekzadeh, A. N., Mbaba, M., & Boone, C. A. (2022). Ending the HIV Epidemic for All, Not Just Some: Structural Racism as a Fundamental but Overlooked Social-Structural Determinant of the US HIV Epidemic. *Current Opinion in HIV and AIDS*, 17(2), 40–45. https://doi.org/10.1097/COH.0000000000000724

Braunstein, S. L., Kersanske, L., Torian, L. V., Lazar, R., & Harriman, G. (2022). Survival among New Yorkers with HIV from 1981 to 2017: Inequities by Race/Ethnicity and Transmission Risk Persist into the Post-HAART Era. *AIDS and Behavior*, 26(1), 284–293. https://doi.org/10.1007/s10461-021-03382-x

Center for Disease Control (CDC). (2018). HIV Prevention and Care Outcomes. www.cdc.gov/hiv/pdf/library/slidesets/cdc-hiv-prevention-and-care-outcomes-2018.pdf. Accessed February 17, 2024.

Community HIV/AIDS Training and Technical Assistance. (2018). Ryan White HIV/AIDS Program, Part A: Planning Council Primer. https://targethiv.org/sites/default/files/file-upload/resources/Primer_June2018.pdf. Accessed October 31, 2023.

COVID Tracking Project. (2021). *The Atlantic.* https://covidtracking.com/data/state/new-york/race-ethnicity. Accessed February 17, 2024.

Crowe, C. & Rosenn, B. (2023). Strengthening NYC's Nonprofits by Reducing Administrative Burdens. https://nycfuture.org/research/reducing-administrative-burdens-on-nonprofits. Accessed October 30, 2023.

The Denver Principles. (1983). https://data.unaids.org/pub/externaldocument/2007/gipa1983denverprinciples_en.pdf. Accessed February 17, 2024.

Freire, P. (1995). *Pedagogy of the Oppressed.* Chicago, IL: Continuum Publishing.

Gaycities. (2011). New York City Department of Health: Its Never Just HIV. www.youtube.com/watch?v=dW0Xw7OOEUI. Accessed October 30, 2023.

HIV.Gov. (2023). Ending the HIV Epidemic Overview. www.hiv.gov/federal-response/ending-the-hiv-epidemic/overview/. Accessed February 17, 2024.

HIV Health and Human Services Planning Council of New York. (2019). *Psycho-social Support Service Directive for People of Transgender, Intersex, Non-Binary and Non-Conforming (TGINBNC) Experience.* https://nyhiv.org/wp-content/uploads/2020/03/TGNB-PSS-Directive_7-25-19_PC-Approved.pdf. Accessed October 28, 2023.

HIV Health and Human Services Planning Council of New York (2021a). *Framing Directive.* https://nyhiv.org/wp-content/uploads/2022/03/Framing-Directive_PC-Approved-12-16-21.pdf. Accessed October 28, 2023.

HIV Health and Human Services Planning Council of New York (2021b). Oral Health Care Service Directive. https://nyhiv.org/wp-content/uploads/2021/05/NYC-Oral-Health-Directive_IOC_PC-Approved.pdf. Accessed October 28, 2023.

HIV Health and Human Services Planning Council of New York (2021c). *Directive for Aging People with HIV.* https://nyhiv.org/wp-content/uploads/2022/01/Directive-for-Aging-PWH_PC-Approved-10-28-21.pdf. Accessed February 17, 2024.

Horn, T. (2010). "It's Never Just HIV" Campaign Divides AIDS Activists. *Poz.Com.* www.poz.com/blog/nycs-public-service. Accessed February 17, 2024.

HRSA Ryan White HIV/AIDS Program. (2023). *Part A: Grants to Eligible Metropolitan and Transitional Grant Areas. The Health Resources and Services Administration's (HRSA) Ryan White HIV/AIDS Program (RWHAP).* https://ryanwhite.hrsa.gov/sites/default/files/ryanwhite/resources/program-factsheet-part.pdf. Accessed February 17, 2024.

Laurencin, C. T., Murdock, C. J., Laurencin, L., & Christensen, D. M. (2018). HIV/AIDS and the African-American Community 2018: A Decade Call to Action. *Journal of Racial and Ethnic Health Disparities*, 5(3), 449–458. https://doi.org/10.1007/s40615-018-0491-0

Livingston, R. (2020). How to Promote Racial Equity in the Workplace: A Five Step Plan. *Harvard Business Review.* https://hbr.org/2020/09/how-to-promote-racial-equity-in-the-workplace. Accessed February 17, 2024.

Millett, G., Peterson, J. L., Flores, S. A., Hart, T. A., Jeffries, W. L., Wilson, P. A., Rourke, S. B., Heilig, C. M., Elford, J., Fenton, K. A., & Remis, R. S. (2012). Comparisons of Disparities and Risks of HIV Infection in Black and Other Men Who Have Sex with Men in Canada, UK, and USA: A Meta-analysis. *The Lancet*, 380(9839), 341–348. https://doi.org/10.1016/S0140-6736(12)60899-X

Mineo, L. (2021). Racial Wealth Gap May Be a Key to Other Inequities: A Look at How and Why We Got There and What We Can Do About It. Unequal: A Series on Race and Injustice in America. *Harvard Gazette.* https://news.harvard.edu/gazette/story/2021/06/racial-wealth-gap-may-be-a-key-to-other-inequities/. Accessed February 17, 2024.

Moreno, J. L. (1978). *Who Shall Survive? Foundations of Sociometry, Group Psychotherapy, and Sociodrama.* University of California, CA: Beacon House.

NYC Health. (2016a). *Race to Justice Action Kit.* www1.nyc.gov/assets/doh/downloads/pdf/dpho/race-to-justice-action-kit-how-to-use-kit.pdf. Accessed February 17, 2024.

NYC Health. (2016b). HIV: Undetectable Equals Untransmittable (U=U). www.nyc.gov/site/doh/providers/health-topics/hiv-u-u.page#. Accessed October 30, 2023.

NYC Health. (2017). *Community Engagement Framework.* www1.nyc.gov/assets/doh/downloads/pdf/che/community-engagement-framework.pdf. Accessed October 28, 2023.

NYC Health. (2021). *HIV Surveillance Annual Report.* www.nyc.gov/assets/doh/downloads/pdf/dires/hiv-surveillance-annualreport-2021.pdf. Accessed October 30, 2023.

NYC Mayor's Office for Economic Opportunity. (2020). *An Economic Profile of Immigrants in New York City 2017: Results from NYC Opportunity's Experimental Population Estimate. February 2020.* www.nyc.gov/site/opportunity/reports/immigrant-economic-profile.page. Accessed February 17, 2024.

Okun, T. (2021). White Supremacy Culture. www.whitesupremacyculture.info. Accessed October 30, 2023.

Spade, D. (2020) *Mutual Aid: Building Solidarity During This Crisis.* London and New York: Verso.

Suluaiman, A. (2020). Stigma & Bias in Healthcare: The Obstacles, Consequences and Changes Needed. Foundation for Healthcare Quality. www.qualityhealth.org/wpsc/2020/08/17/stigma-bias-in-healthcare-the-obstacles-consequences-and-changes-needed/. Accessed October 28, 2023.

Undoing Racism: Peoples' Institute for Survival and Beyond (PISAB). (n.d.). Our Principles. https://pisab.org/our-principles/. Accessed October 28, 2023.

United States Census Bureau. (2021). Quick Facts: New York City, New York. www.census.gov/quickfacts/newyorkcitynewyork. Accessed February 17, 2024.

The White House. (2021). *National HIV/AIDS Strategy for the United States 2022–2025.* www.whitehouse.gov/wp-content/uploads/2021/11/National-HIV-AIDS-Strategy.pdf. Accessed February 17, 2024.

Wortsman, P. (2015). Alumni Profile: Mary T. Bassett'79: A Champion of Health Equality at the Helm of the NYC Department of Health. Columbia University, School of Medicine. www.columbiamedicinemagazine.org/alumni-news-notes/fall-2015/alumni-profile-mary-t-bassett'79. Accessed February 17, 2024.

Chapter 9

Contemporary Applications of Jung's Method of Active Imagination in Activist Arts-Based Research and Psychodrama

Robin McCoy Brooks

A Crisp Introduction

C. G. Jung claimed that his method of active imagination held the potential to creatively transform the psyche-social development of the individual. I am interested in extending Jung's vision for his method into broader collective contexts that are relevant to psychology today. To this end, I first address the personal and historical conditions that compelled Jung to discover active imagination while elaborating the dynamism of its process. From this historical background, I explore various approaches to contemporary research and group psychology that embrace Jung's methodology. I begin by illustrating how active imagination has influenced the development of my professional writing process. Moreover, Gloria Anzaldúa's innovative approach to professional writing accessed active imagination to facilitate social activism. Her activist arts-based research continues to ignite Latinx feminist philosophical discourse today. Jungian scholar Susan Rowland has rigorously argued that Jung's discovery of active imagination is, at its core, arts-based research (ABR), thus creating a new category of ABR she terms Jungian arts-based research (JABR) (Rowland & Weishaus, 2021). Finally, I examine and illustrate how Jacob Levey Moreno's mutual aid approach to group psychology and Jung's method of active imagination extend and refine the efficacy of the other. Moreno's form of group psychotherapy can also be considered a form of activist arts-based research.

Introducing Jung's Method of Active Imagination

Carl Gustav Jung (1875–1961) began to experience the agonizing effects of "soul-loss" following his break with Freud and the onset of World War I (Hillman & Shamdasani, 2013, pp. 24, 67). Lethargy, mercurial moodiness, and a series of significant dreams compelled him to engage in a process of self-experimentation based on the natural function of imagination and the desire to heal himself from within. From 1913 to 1916, Jung experimented with a number of meditative processes that facilitated his engagement with his unconscious

DOI: 10.4324/9781003386339-13

mind while maintaining a self-reflective (conscious) stance. In this way, he explored his inner landscapes and engaged with the fantasies, visions, and other symbolic forms of psyche that spontaneously emerged (Jung, 1916/1957/1972, pp. 131–193). The psyche's artifacts come to us, in other words. We do not imagine them or make them up. At best, we receive, engage with, and interpret them.

The Red Book editor Sonu Shamdasani describes three levels of Jung's psychological process, culminating in what today is known as *The Red Book Liber Novus* (Shamdasani, 2009, p. 33). After each session, Jung carefully recorded the visionary encounters that emerged as he experienced them in black leather-bound journals. Then, he stepped back to obtain a conceptual perspective that allowed him to interpret his experiences. Last, he laboriously transferred selections from the black journals to a red leather-bound journal (*The Red Book*) and meticulously illustrated sections with a series of well-rendered paintings and mandalas. Later, Jung refined and named his self-healing practice *active imagination* (Jung, 1935/1989, paras. 390–415).

Jung was interested in attuning to the expressions of psychic energy (unconscious activity) that we traditionally think of as reflected in dream work, fantasy, and the intensification of symptoms (Jung, 1928/1981, pp. 19–20). His method contained three primary states, simply described as letting the unconscious arise and then coming to terms with it by bringing its significance into consciousness (Chodorow, 1997; Swan-Foster, 2018). Coming to terms with what emerges involves *amplifying* the images, symptoms, experiences, and so on. Amplification, as I use it, includes both personal association and researching from sources that are external to the individual's associations, with the intention of making meaning from them.

For example, I recall a patient's dream image that I shared with Wolfgang Giegerich in a supervision session. I asked Giegerich to demonstrate how I might "amplify" a dream scene that portrayed a lifeless man, stretched out on a table in the center of an empty room. His naked body was partially covered with a sheet. Upon hearing the dream, Giegerich ran out of the consultation room (we were in his home) to one of his three libraries, returning with a large art book. He opened the book to a reproduction of a painting by Italian Renaissance artist Andrea Mantegna, entitled "The Lamentation of Christ." Perhaps you are familiar with this painting. The dead Christ figure is laying on his back on a hard surface, with a cloth covering the lower part of his body. Because of the perspective, I was at first drawn to his feet dominating the lower center of the canvas. However, my eye was immediately directed to his genitals. This shockingly realistic perspective gave me the impression of actually being in a morgue. The patient's dream image became viscerally alive for me. He was impotent, powerless, and dead to himself, I thought. For Jung, Christ was a symbol of the self. A "dead" Christ image, if I relied on Giegerich's amplification, revealed the severity of the patient's dissociation from his depths. He had no internal rudder. In later sessions, the patient began to talk about his uselessness in the world. Amplification has the potential to open new areas of understanding that are either unconscious or hidden.

The last step of active imagination involves taking responsibility, which leads to, in Jung's words, "a new level of being, a new situation" (Jung, 1916/1957/1972, para. 189). Eventually, the dreamer, noted above, would develop a capacity to bear a *truth about his uselessness*. After a long and complicated series of events, he began to identify a *truth about his desire*. This would lead eventually to the realization that he could purposefully share certain capabilities he had with the world. The various fetishes and addictions that he had formerly misperceived as objects of desire faded away as new, and less complex versions, emerged.[1]

Jung developed a synthetic method of interpretating unconscious activity (with the patient) with the aim of discovering a solution to a symptom or dilemma (Jung, 1912/1957/1967). He differentiated two kinds of thinking that were a basis for his synthetic method: *directed and non-directed*.[2] The process of non-directed thinking is inwardly directed, and is facilitated by dropping into an often non-verbal space, attuning to bodily sensations and symptoms, strange or peculiar dreams, emotion, imagination, creative or destructive impulses, utterances, vision, fleeting fragments of fantasy, a nothingness or lack, and so on (Jung, 1912/1957/1967). These spaces may open to us in sleep, spontaneously in group and individual therapy, or at a stop light, for example when we are exposed to a destabilizing psychical and/or real-world event.

Directed thinking was the companion process to non-directed thinking that Jung proposed. Directed thinking is an objective, linear, and empirically based process where the imprint of non-directed material works its way into verbal expression and possibly action, as we saw with the patient I described above through the amplification of his dream work. Put another way, the function of the synthetic method facilitates a transition from one psychic condition to another by means of mutual confrontation of opposites, as Jung had first discovered from his active imagination inquiries in *The Red Book* (Jung, 1954/1975, p. 489). Jung named the overall process the *transcendent function*, which he viewed as a *process and a method* at the same time. Building a capacity to bear the tension of opposing positions, without siding with one against the other, has the potential to build inter and intrapsychic rapport, and can transform a particular personal or collective situation. Jung named the procedural method of engaging opposing positions within one's psyche *active imagination*.

A Collective Loss of Eros

Jungian scholar Susan Rowland concludes that *The Red Book* was generated from a profound rupture in Jung's psyche, leading him to visions that revealed a plethora of splits, not only within his personal psyche *but also* within the psyche of Western modernity (Rowland & Weishaus, 2021, p. 99). *The Red Book* editor Sonu Shamdasani notes that in 1914, there was a shift in Jung's journal writing when he realized his visionary figures were literally, or symbolically, imbricated with culture and, most auspiciously, the outbreak of the Great War on the European continent (Hillman & Shamdasani, 2013, p. 130; Jung, 2012, p. 474; Brooks, 2023). *The questions we grapple with, Jung surmised, arise from a part of our personal and collective experience we are neglecting* (Hillman & Shamdasani, 2013, p. 24).

To illustrate this important point further, I turn to a passage from one of Jung's grisly visions. Jung encounters a lifeless child in the rubble of a dystopian landscape. A mysterious cloaked figure asks him to atone for the child's death *by eating a piece of her liver*. Furthermore, he must actually cut the liver piece out of her tiny corpse (Jung, 2009, p. 290). Horrified, Jung resists. *He* is *not* the murderer, he rants, demanding to know who is giving him such an order. The figure responds by telling Jung that *he* is the child's soul, and the child needs atonement that he must do, for her sake. *"You share this guilt ... because you are a man and a man has committed this deed"* (Jung, 2009, p. 290). With this astonishing discovery, Jung sinks down and surrenders. He accepts his culpability. After completing the horrific deed, the mysterious figure throws back their veil, revealing that *she* is "his soul." In Jung's next narrative breath, having performed a healing ritual that parallels the Catholic mass, he identifies the sacrificial child as the divine offspring, of the mother, of his soul (Jung, 2009, p. 291, f. 151; Brooks, 2023 pp. 84–85).[3]

From this and other visionary experiences, Jung concluded that the dead of human history demanded atonement for unresolved violence, murder, wrongdoing, contempt, or *lives that were incomplete*, in such a way that reverberated with his *"present incompleteness"* (Jung, 2012, p. 346). On this phenomenon, he later clarified:

> ... when a problem which is at bottom personal, and therefore apparently subjective, coincides with the external events that contain the same psychological elements as personal conflict, it is suddenly transformed into a general question embracing the whole of society. In this way, a personal problem acquires a dignity it lacked hitherto, since the inner discord always has something humiliating and degrading about it.
>
> (Jung, 1971, para. 119)

Jung discovered that the forgotten dead of human history resonated with the parts of his personal psyche that he was also ignoring. To both, he must make amends. He followed the advice of a soul figure: "turn to the dead, listen [to them] and accept them with love," and actively engage them with a courage and tenderness born of eros – the "law of love" (Jung, 2012, pp. 344, 346–347).[4] From where do these images arise, the soul figures, the lifeless child? Later, Jung would make a distinction between the personal and collective psyche, yet in this passage, these figures appear to be personal (subjective and personal history) *and* archetypal (a collective unconscious).

"The dead haunt," Rowland and Weishaus note, because they have been cut out of historical memory, due to a collective loss of *Eros* (love) (Rowland & Weishaus, 2021, pp. 94–95). Building on Rowland and Weishaus's statement, if *Eros* becomes estranged in the collective psyche, and I believe it has in today's era, then cultural care is not comprehended, valued, or concretized in either the subjective *or* collective realms. This dynamic is reflected in how we structure all levels of our society, becoming vulnerable to societal processes of *elimination* (genocide, exile), *marginalization* (of otherness), and *disempowerment* (slavery) (Hinton, 2011; Brooks, 2016). Splitting off from self and humanitarian care contributes to collective atrophy, *losing our minds*, and we are in danger of becoming a "soulless herd animal" (Jung, 1998, p. 248).[5]

The collective loss of *Eros* is, in my opinion, one of the central concerns in contemporary society, as it was in Jung's era. Our contemporary political moment is defined by escalating and uncontained crises. Governmental policies, and strategies that are designed to attend to these looming crises, remain grossly inadequate. Social injustices, climate degradation, and healthcare mismanagement continue to ignore and exacerbate harm (Hartman, 2021). Certainly, this is a grave concern for us all.

Jung did not consider social transformation to be an *immediate* agenda for psychoanalysis, although his work foreshadowed later psychosocial contributions put forth by luminaries of group and community psychology, elaborated in Chapter 3. Nevertheless, he understood that the questions and conflicts we grapple with arise from both our subjective and collective experiences that we are neglecting. This includes the effects of real and concrete events of our era.[6]

Psychology has become a palliative intervention attending to the symptoms of collective carelessness and not the cause. Mainstream remedies do not draw on our full potential, as human beings, to care and radically orient ourselves towards creating a kind of world we can fall in love with. The blatant bias against the viability of group psychology, for example, ignores how embedded we are in group life in all facets of our profession. We conduct research, teach, learn, participate, supervise, consult, and convene in groups regularly, often without any formal training. Furthermore, we generally do not consider how many cultures within the United States thrive within collectivism, as a direct result of connection to community, as described in Chapter 2 (Musso, 2023).[7]

Jung's method of active imagination was intended to be a self-healing tool for patients conducted outside of individual therapy sessions. What draws me to Jungian psychology is a shared belief that each of us has healing wisdom within our being. Developing strategies and practices that build intra-psychical rapport is one of the aims of psychodynamic therapy, and certainly active imagination. We will see in the last section of this chapter how Jacob Levy Moreno, founder of group psychotherapy, would extend the self-healing capacity of the individual into a group's capacity to heal each other, but I am getting ahead of myself.

Traditional Jungian psychology (and psychoanalysis in general) remains focused on the individual. Jungian analysts, Jungian arts-based researchers, Jungian art therapists, psychodynamically oriented therapists, hypnotherapists, sand play therapists, child play therapists, body-oriented workers, psychedelic-assisted therapists, academic researchers, and psychodrama group therapists (to name a few) are creatively adopting aspects of active imagination in individual and clinical and academic group work (Stephenson, 2014; Swan-Foster, 2018; Attinello, 2023; Rowland, 2023).

In the following sections, I discuss how active imagination has been creatively used in a variety of contemporary applications as means of extending the relevancy of depth psychology. I begin with a personal illustration of how the practice of active imagination has contributed to the development of my professional writing.

Writing In Between

My father died as I was climbing Mt. Rainier with Quest, in 1999. As a child, I believed that my father was the smartest person in my world. He excelled in math, was an intelligence officer, and earned a Ph.D. in political science during the Cold War. My mother was a lieutenant in the army and met my father while caring for his war injuries. Her magnificent mind was later used to raise a family and support my father's career. While I was encouraged to think independently, my interests were vastly other to those of my pragmatic parents.

When my father died, I started having spontaneous and reoccurring images of a forest savagely burning to the ground.[8] I painted the fireball, over and over. At the same time, I fiercely started cleaning out my closets. I divorced my husband and became a single parent. I was sloughing off old skin, lost, in a white-out ... familiar landmarks are gone. I am off trail and drop into the heightened sensibility of the animal world. I become a little animal. In the mountains, my body/mind moves stealthily through a timeless wilderness. Sleeping near the Ohanapecosh glacier, on Mt. Rainier, I dream of deer and awaken, literally, to deer hoof prints circling my head. While driving, I am visited by reoccurring visual flashes of running with deer, bright sunlight flickering through trees. I recall a crystal vase with the Goddess Artemis etched on its side. I dig it out of storage, suddenly remembering that my mother gave it to me before she died. My heart cracks wide open. My mother had knowledge of my core – before I did, now 20 years after her death. I had killed off Artemis and now she was returning to me, demanding to be heard. I start painting her – running with my deer companion, holding a bow in one hand. What am I hunting?

I was internally hemorrhaging, divided in two, a kind of half being, fractured between two kinds of desire. The fantasy-driven Artemis is libidinally animated – fearless in the wilderness. She is alive in her animality ... hunting.

Who or what is she hunting? Is hers a cupid's arrow or is she seeking prey? She sees a figure on the hill, aims, and with a whoosh, shoots. The body thuds heavily to the ground. Stealthy, she moves through the trees. Arriving on the scene, she kneels to the ground. The body has fallen on a bed of giant ferns, a soft landing from the heights of abstraction (ideas). The head moves and slowly turns to her now. Their eyes lock. Who are you? – is wordlessly conveyed between them. And ... what do you want from me? A new relationship strangely animates something between them, shared, but not their own. New life flashes up and is directed back and forth, from the mindless body to the bloodless mind – a mutual transfusion that spawns a new and enigmatic field of possibility.

Between inexplicable pre-cognitive impulse (Artemis/Eros) and careful logic (Logos) arises a new possibility. I began to recognize aspects of myself that I had killed off in my professional writing (and in general). These aspects included my creative energies, imagination, in-spirited presence, love of nature, and animal body/heart. Personalizing Eros requires that I do not kill off my love of theory either and ability to rigorously engage its abstractions (Logos/mind/spirit). I struggle with my psychical contradictions in every page of this book.

Jung would call the transaction between the Artemis figure and mind (Logos) *coniunctio*—an alchemical symbol of a union between alien substances; a marrying of psychical opposites, from which comes the birth of a new element. Anzaldúa called the new element spiritual power from which spiritual activism becomes possible. Spiritual activism is the child of such a union. Moreno would direct me to put my process into action on the psychodramatic stage. We move our resources into action and share them with others, in nine thousand ways that contribute to making our world one we love and love in.

In 2002, I knew it was time to pursue becoming a Jungian analyst. The intensity of the AIDS crisis was lessening with the discovery of antiviral treatments. I was being released from the gravity of AIDS and thrown to the ground. I began training in 2004, stimulated by a process of de-idealizing Jung and psychoanalysis in general. I started to challenge my transferential relationship to patriarchy, teasing out how Freud, or Jung's theories of mind, offered little to clarify my experiences of group process or what had happened in the early Quest years that amalgamated a whole community towards social change. The hierarchical rigidity of my training institute baffled me in stark contrast to my envelopment in a mutual aid community.

Psychoanalytic institutes are infamously known for splitting apart because of the inability to comprehend and work through complex group dynamics. Traditional institutes are rigidly hierarchical. Psychoanalysis is generally critiqued for its arrogant attitude and exclusivity, perpetuated by claiming to hold certainties about the "true" nature of human suffering. This attitude is accompanied by hierarchical interpretive practices that seem to always know the *subject* better than they know themselves (Billig, 1997; Wetherell, 2003; Frosh & Baraitser, 2008; Brooks, 2019; Saban, 2019).

Under the tutelage of several analyst mentors, especially Ladson Hinton, Michael Horne, Wolfgang Giegerich, and Bob Stuckey, my mind opened to the history of ideas, giving me a cross-disciplinary context from which I began to think expansively about how the self and social psyche co-engaged with a public realm. This opened a door. I was inspired to learn the conceptual language systems of several psychoanalytic and philosophical traditions. I wrote many scholarly papers, chapters, and a book. I was finding my way through obscure theoretical depictions of psyche by retranslating key concepts into phenomenological terms. I was and continue to be thrilled by the abstraction of ideas and my rigorous ability to grind out new understanding.

Nevertheless, my writing was often bloodless, gripped by intellectual convention. I adopted a publishable academic writing style and psychoanalytic lexicon that excluded readers outside of my esoteric puniverse. While I no longer was running with the deer, I had new intellectual companions and was building my own library.

The Red Book was first released in 2009 while I was finishing psychoanalytic training. Remarkably, the *RB* is stripped of the confusing, bloodless, metaphysical reification that Jung later developed in the *Collected Works*. Jung's contributions to understanding human experience in my view are many. However, their principal significance became more accessible to me through his personal accounting of nuanced transformations that occurred within his primitive self. These occurred in relationship with the spontaneous production of visions, fantasies, and images that erupted from his personal and collective psyche—that reservoir of world history, culture, and myth.

These passages reinvigorated my relationship with Jung's later scholarship, opening a window into my own. How was my internalized misogyny and self-erasure intersecting with ideologies inculcated by dominant sectors of society *and* mainstream theories and practices within the broader field of psychology today, including depth psychology? My psyche was gristle for my own teeth, in tandem with cultural norms that maintain social injustice at all levels of being. Why, I wondered, are the scholarly voices of women not adequately represented in the training curriculum? Where are the queer, non-white, and international voices of Jungian analysts and scholars? How can analytical psychology help advance social change and political activism if we don't have adequate tools to relate to each other? How can we broaden our theoretical and clinical frame to include the psychosocial realities, group processes, and the concrete world?

Until I started writing this book with my psychoanalytic colleagues seven years ago, I rarely discussed that I work with groups or have extensive training in psychodrama and group psychotherapy. Once I referred to my experiences with Quest, in a training seminar; I forget the context. I suspect my psyche was erupting from a stranglehold I had been maintaining since becoming a candidate because of a long-held bias against group therapy (see Chapter 3). Michael Horne, the seminar leader, looked at me with amusement and remarked with a wave of his hand that he didn't know *how* I managed to handle all of those transferences. How do any of us manage to remember who we are amidst all of the transferences that hang in the air like unmetabolized sewage? I think his question emblematically describes the perception of the impenetrable gap between individual psychology and group psychology, alluding to how little we understand transferential phenomena on a collective scale.

I started reading the radical works of Gloria Anzaldúa (1942–2004). Anzaldúa was influenced by and extended Jung's method of active imagination into her own self-writing practice she named *Autohistoria-teoría.*[9] She wrote with powerful and interpretive freedom, describing a recursive "path of two-way movement – a going deep into the self and expanding out into the world," —a simultaneous recreation of the self *and* a reconstruction of society (Anzaldúa, 1981/2014, p. 208).

Unlike Jung, Anzaldúa linked personal healing directly with social activism. She did not separate the personal unconscious from the collective, sociopolitical, and ancestral forces that invisibilized her spiritual existance (Anzaldúa, 1987, p. 59).

Had our paths crossed at the University of Texas when I was in art school, I wondered? Probably not, as I was oblivious to my white privilege, living in an all-white dorm in the 1970s, shamefully complicit in her erasure as a person, and my own. The viscerality of Anzaldúa's poetry gutted me in *Borderlands* (1987) 35 years later. For nights, I had nightmares. I recall wrestling with greater opponents and waking up in sweat-soaked sheets. Her work deepened my own, pulling me into the division between my animal body and in-spirited knowledge, between traditional and arts-based research genres, between group and individual psychology.

Concurrently, I felt the urge to paint again. Presently, I am painting a large image of Mt. Rainier on the walls of my living room. Why not let our creativity spill out into our living spaces, generated from existential anguish and love? In a state of spiritual searching, Moreno once claimed to have written poems on his walls, imagining God was speaking to him in the here and now (Moreno, 1971). What I was searching for cannot be contained in a frame, genre, body, or mind. Its erratic and enigmatic expressions need open spaces to roam freely.

My personal academic writing process is often excruciating, wrought with paralyzing bouts of anxiety and feelings of inferiority.[10] My husband, Ted, is a creative and writes with me. Side by side on the couch on the boat with our animals, or in our room-less home. We accompany each other through our separate and twin anxieties, pushing through. My son Elliott and niece Barbi are writing their dissertations—companions across the country. My little brother Paul died suddenly two weeks ago, his dissertation almost completed. Writing this sentence pulls me into the blackness of his unspeakable loss. This book is fueled by unspeakable loss and the knowledge of a kind of love that breaks through the dead of winter. The avalanche lily.

Anxiety fertilizes the ground for the possibility of a new deliverance. Anxiety signals an encounter with radical otherness, according to Jacques Lacan (2014, p. 207). Encountering the blank page (wall, screen, or face) often exposes me to a fundamental void. If I can bear the libidinal intensity without fleeing, or going up in flames, nothing may open to something else and demands I relate to it. Sometimes nothing comes. I struggled for months, for example writing and rewriting the first section of this chapter before I realized my true challenge was to write from the intersection of conceptual (thought) and prose. To move back and forth between the banks of a flooding river and dried out river-bed … where formlessness incarnates itself, raw, vulnerable, skinless—seeking new expression.[11]

Gloria Anzaldúa, Autohistoria-teoría, and Spiritual Activism

Anzaldúa was a philosopher, poet, author, and queer feminist of color who explored aesthetic forms of knowledge production. She creatively reimagined Jung's notion of the "transcendent function" into a concept she termed *neptantla* (Anzaldúa, 2015, p. 127). Neptantla is a term that means the space "in between" taken from Nahuatl, the Aztec language, from which Anzaldúa (1987) claimed Indigenous ancestry as a sixth generation mexicanos from the Rio Grande Valley of South Texas. Neptantla represents a painful and potentially transformational inter and intra-psychical space, where opposing realities converge, conflict, and metamorphize (Anzaldúa, 2015, pp. 242–244). Anzaldúa elaborates in theoretical prose:

> Some point on the way to new consciousness, we will have to leave the opposite between two mortal combatants somehow healed so that we are on *both shores at once* and, at once, *see through serpent and eagle eyes.* Or perhaps we will decide to disengage from the dominant culture, write it off altogether as a lost cause, and cross the border into a wholly new and separate territory. Or we might consider another route. The possibilities are numerous once we decide to act and not react.
>
> (Anzaldúa, 1987, pp. 100–101, my emphasis)

Seeing through "serpent and eagle eyes" is a metaphor for newly acquired knowledge that contributes to novel understanding and action amidst a field of contradictions and ambivalences without psychical splitting. It is the "third eye" that *simultaneously* looks inward and outward, as a result of reflective consciousness (Anzaldúa, 2015, p. 120, 2000, p. 178).

The "eagle" and "serpent" are symbols inspired by the Aztec goddess *Coatlicue* whose image first terrifyingly entered Anzaldúa's psyche in a terrible nightmare when she was three years old (Anzaldúa, 1987, pp. 68–73). *Coatlicue* was the Aztec mountain earth goddess of birth and death. She describes how biases in

Westernized, Chicana culture sought to kill off her psyche/spiritual experiences. "Like many Indians and Mexicans, I did not deem my psychic experiences real. I denied their occurrences and let my inner senses atrophy" (Anzaldúa, 1987, p. 59).

Anzaldúa's writing intersects the geo/political/historical colonization of Mexico with the psyche/social oppression of the female, Chicano, queer, psyche that she seeks to heal throughout her work.

Thus, to be "on both shores at once," thereby seeing through "serpent and eagle eyes," requires that we live within constantly shifting border cultures in between opposing perspectives and realities so that a state of being *beyond binary thinking* arises. We build a transformational tolerance, in other words, for our contradictory and conflated identities that arise in geographies, political narratives, languages, race, sexualities, religions, uncritically held histories, genders, and so on. "Speaking across the divide," or on both sides at once, she called *mestizaje*, the *new mestiza* consciousness and later *conocimiento*—a word in Spanish that means knowledge (Anzaldúa, 1987, 2015).[12] *Conocimiento* is described this way:

> If you are tender with yourself, you can be tender to others … The spiritual practice of *conocimiento*, such as praying, breathing deeply, meditating, writing – dropping down into yourself, through the skin and muscles and tendons, down deep into the bones; marrow where your soul is ballast – enabled you to defuse the negative … and other killer of the spirit. Spirituality becomes a port you moor in all storms.
>
> (Anzaldúa, 2015, pp. 154–155)

Anzaldúa's self-writing practice incorporated arts-based practices to tap into spiritual knowledge, in contrast to collectively conditioned narratives that violently erase human diversity, dignity, ancestry, tradition, history, and well-being. On this she states:

> What you live through and the knowledge you infer from experience is subjective. Intuitive knowing, unmediated by mental constructs – what inner eye, heart, and gut tell you – is the closest you come to direct knowledge (gnosis) of the world, and this experience of reality is partial, too.
>
> (Anzaldúa, 2015, pp. 119–120)

The first step to acquiring "direct" knowledge of the world and our place in it, she claims, begins with opening our senses and consciously inhabiting our bodies within its surroundings, sensations, intuitions, emotional reactivities, instincts, and lived experiences, as well as engaging with the creative arts, especially writing, but also making art, dancing, teaching, meditation, and spiritual activism (Anzaldúa, 2015, pp. 117, 120).[13] The parallels to Jung's method of opening to his depths in active imagination are obvious.

Clearly, Anzaldúa's genre of writing was a vividly *relational* form of personal and cultural autobiography, generated by *re*writing narratives accessed through historical references, ancestorial heritage, theoretical prose, memoir, cultural myth, cultural critique, imaginal elaboration, metaphor, poetry, and the linguistic movement between English, Castilian Spanish, North Mexican dialect, Tex-Mex, and occasional *Nahuad* (Anzaldúa, 1987). She self-identified as an academic *and* spiritual activist (Anzaldúa, 2015). She did not create the term spiritual activism but introduced it into post-colonial scholarship (Crowley, 2011). Knowledge transformation was a decolonizing process in that her writing style was completely embodied and politically subversive (Keating, 2015, p. xxiv). Her works purposefully disrupted and challenged existing power structures that limited and constrained women and women of color by transforming what *was missing from dominating discourses* into new theoretical models through her writing (Anzaldúa, 2015, p. 7).[14]

Anzaldúa put her writing into action by engaging in reflective dialogue with others and building coalitional spaces (*nepantla*) with a shared vision of ending multiple oppressions (not just one's own) in the coexistence of shared concerns (Pitts, 2021, p. 155). She sought allies, in other words, with the intention of co-creating "spiritual/political" communities that both encouraged healing and mobilized social change. She writes:

> To be in conocimiento with another person or group is to share knowledge, pool resources, meet each other, compare liberation struggles and social movements' histories, share how we confront institutional power, and process and heal wounds. In conocimiento, we seek input from communities so as not to fall into elite collective, isolated cells that widen the chasm between ... politics and grassroots activism ... solidarity work demands a global, all-embracing vision ...we apply what we learn to all of our daily activities, to our relationships with ourselves, with others with the environment, with nature.
>
> (Anzaldúa, 2015, p. 91)

The link between Anzaldúa's self-writing practice, personal authenticity, spiritual activism, and a mutual aid approach to sharing her work is clear. She sought mutual exchange with a shared desire for personal healing and social change. Coalitional spaces were collaboratively created and resources were pooled and shared in order to move towards a shared liberatory vision.

Arts-Based Research (ABR)

The arts have been creatively applied towards understanding and communicating human experience since time immemorial. The recent history of arts-based research methods, however, is arguably varied. The term ABR was coined in the early 1990s by art educator Elliott Eisner (Rolling, 2013, p. 3). Today, ABR is emerging as a major methodological research practice materialized through art practices such as writing forms (academic and creative writing), poetry, digital art, laser art, machinal (robot) constructions, architectural art (such as in Burning Man), music-making, computer games, painting, sculpture, photography, film-making, illustrated novels, performance arts, and what is yet to be created.[15]

ABR is an alternative to traditionally held research approaches and attempts to transform and critique status quo understandings of what research is (Pearse, 1983, p. 161). Scientific research generally separates the researcher from the research by relying on quantitative methods that objectify subjectivity as a means of verifying subsequent claims. They become *uni-focused* models of reality, derived and applied universally, with the understanding that we are all alike. This is one of the major critiques of Western-centric theories and practices that have been conceived from the perspective of the colonizer, as discussed in Chapter 2.

The *multi-model* approach to theory building in ABR values a plurality of approaches from other disciplines that allow us to consider the diverse and provisional aspect of being human, which is lost in uni-focused methods. The more nuanced understandings of the intersectional effects of race, class, gender, sexuality, disability, religion, ethnicity, culture, genetic heritage, socio/political landscape, and neurodiversity (to name a few) of individual or collective reality are less considered in mainstream psychological uni-focused paradigms. Graham poignantly discusses how these uni-focused models of care contribute to oppressive practices in mental health public program administration in Chapter 8. Additionally, scientific knowledge is divided (siloed) into academic disciplines, falling into siloed hierarchies and making multi-disciplinary conversations difficult, if not impossible.

The purpose of ABR is to build theory through a mediated interpretation of materials, languages, social contexts, and experiences that shape and clarify the researcher's unfolding purpose. By its very nature, ABR is an inclusive research method that values different ways of understanding our experiences, or even what knowledge is. Art is seen as a "reflexive system for thinking improvisationally manifested as a heterogeneous continuum of experiential learning possibilities," in contrast to proving certainties (Rolling, 2013, p. 13).

There is no single definition of ABR, as the field is as diversely described as its multiplicitous expressions. James Haywood Rolling, Jr., however, identifies four modes of ABR that often overlap within a project. He states:

> [ABR is] ... The multisystemic application of interactive, analytical, synthetic, *critical-activist*, or improvisatory creative cognitive processes and artistic practices toward theory-building. Best at addressing questions that can neither be measured with exactitude nor generalized as universally applicable or meaningful in all contexts. Stems directly from a researcher's artistic practice of creative worldview.
>
> (Rolling, 2013, p. 8; my emphasis)

Generally speaking, the *analytical* mode involves thinking in materials; the *synthetic* mode synthesizes or reinterprets multiple narratives/discourses into new understandings; the *critical-activist* inquiry critiques and reinterprets problematic social constructions into new liberatory representations; and the *improvisatory* mode lets the art practice go where it wants across modes (Rolling, 2013, p. 101; Rowland, 2023).

Rolling (2013, p. 108). briefly acknowledges Anzaldúa's work to be a "critical-activist" form of ABR. Critical-activist ABR "produces resistance narratives – counter stories to authoritative grand narratives that are critical, indigenous or local, and anti-oppressive" (Brown & Strega, 2005, in Rolling, 2013, p. 109). Anzaldúa's arts-based research project did not stop with her writing. She created a grassroots social movement by boldly sharing her subjective and theoretical material in reflective dialogue with others in the public domain. Her theoretical works continue to influence Chicanx, Latinx, women of color feminisms, women's studies, queer studies, ethnic studies, and gender studies (Ruiz, 2020; Pitts, 2021). Her research has certainly inspired me and countless other scholars to creatively explore intersectionality within our own research projects.

Critical-activist ABR inquiries interrogate and reinterpret discourses that "dominate, delimit, and distort perceptions and conventions" within our social contexts (Rolling, 2018, p. 506). Anzaldúa radically redirects public attention to what is missing in traditional depictions of the human experience. Against the status quo, she designates what knowledge is and explores through a variety of domains that are neither wholly qualitative nor quantitative, scientific nor artistic, subjective nor objective but are activated "in between" [nepantla space] meanings and methods (Springgay, 2002, p. 106). ABR inquiries recognize arts practices as "twin peaks" alongside scientific practices, yet they erode the borders between both (Rolling, 2013). On this point, Anzaldúa remarks: *"By making certain personal experiences the subject of this study, I also blur the private/public borders"* (Anzaldúa, 2015, p. 6).[16]

Jungian Arts-Based Research (JABR)

Susan Rowland and her husband Joel Weishaus recently wrote a seminal book introducing a new research paradigm named Jungian arts-based research (JARB) (2021). JABR is an extension of ABR, using Jungian ideas and methodologies to provide research strategies such as intuition, synchronicity, amplification, archetypes/collective unconscious, and active imagination, to name a few (Clarke, 2023; Nikkel & Tamsen-Trent, 2023).[17] In a later work, Rowland briefly describes JABR as:

> …. doing therapy with the whole world. It means making knowledge through creativity, the imagination and the unknown psyche or the unconscious interacting with the wisdom of the centuries materialized in art traditions … It is formational, in gathering what matters in the artist, and the work,

informational in finding out what is hidden, and transformational in offering new ways of being.

(Rowland, 2023, p. 436)

I find Rowland's work to be *liberatory*, invigorating, timely, and intuitively familiar, and at its base a form of activism. How could doing therapy with the "whole world" not be radical? JABR is an alternative research paradigm designed to generate knowledge that unites artistic expression, spirit, mind, and body. Rowland's work explodes with relevance in the Jungian world by giving space for a multiplicity of research expressions that itself is subversive. JABR is designed to be shared in a variety of venues such as in virtual and live conferences and performances, which is where I was first introduced to the approach.[18]

Rowland considers Jung's oeuvre to be innately ABR. This is demonstrated through his theories and practices that surpass mainstream psychotherapy because they extend his work into spiritual practice, philosophy, world religion, historical meaning, image, and imagination (Rowland & Weishaus, 2021, pp. 1–25). In the *Handbook of Arts-Based Research*, Cathy Malchiodi acknowledges Freud and Jung as pioneers of ABR because of their innovative inquiry into the unconscious (Malchiodi, 2018, p. 73). *The Red Book* is called a "personal, and seminal example of arts-based research" (Ibid.). Rowland and Weishaus (2021) elaborate on the relevance of the *RB* as ABR by examining the text through Rolling's four genres of ABR described above.

The Red Book was not published in Jung's lifetime because it was not the kind of research he wished to publicly pursue. He never completed the *RB* and belabored what to do with it throughout his lifetime. A century later, his descendants decided to release the volumes for publication, in the care of Jungian scholar Sonu Shamdasani. The significance of the *RB* is cogently described by Shamdasani as a "caesura, [that] opens the possibility of a new era in the understanding of Jung's work today, one that does not end with a conclusion, but the promise of a new beginning" (Shamdasani, 2009, p. 221). This is one of the crowning characteristics of ABR, in that no one owns the meaning of a work and any of us can generate novel meanings about its significance *without limit*.

Jung was critical of war, religion, science, and other dominating cultural and academic discourses in Western modernity that privileged rationality over imagination, intuition, creativity, nature, embodiment, and spiritual presence (1912/1957/1967, *CW 18*, para. 1100). This critique remains relevant today. The direction of his work radically departed from the unifocal materialistic, scientific approaches dominating the emerging field of psychology (then and now) because he positioned the psyche as the core of being and knowing (1912/1957/1967). He later considered *The Red Book* to be a story about a "battle between the world of reality, and the world of the spirit," from which he would clarify and deepen the direction of his psychology (Shamdasani, 2009, p. 213).[19] From this perspective, Jung's *Red Book* is paradigmatically a critical-activist art-based inquiry that became the nucleus for his later works. Jung, however, did not consider social transformation to be an immediate agenda for his psychology, although he understood how individuation was culturally contingent. Contemporary Jungians, in addition to Rowland, are extending aspects of his work into psychosocial studies, as are we with this book (Watkins and Shulman, 2008; Samuels, 2015; Saban, 2020; Lu, 2020; Carpani, 2021; Brooks, 2022; Lu & Yeoman, 2023).

Jung and Moreno

Moreno critiqued a significant oversight in Jung's psychology, which because of its clarity I relay in full:

> We must look for a concept which is so constructed that the objective indication for the existence of this two-way process does not come from a single psyche but from a deeper reality in which the unconscious states of two or several individuals are interlocked with a system of "co-unconscious" states. Jung postulated that every individual has, besides a personal, a collective unconscious. Although the distinction may be useful, it does not help in solving the dilemma described. Jung does not apply the collective unconscious to the concrete collectivities in which people live. There is nothing gained in turning from a personal to a "collective unconscious" if by doing this, the anchorage to the *concrete*, whether individual or group, is lost. Had he [Jung] turned to the group by developing techniques like group psychotherapy or sociodrama, he might have gained a concrete position for his theory of the collective unconscious, but, as it is, he underplayed the individual anchorage but did not establish a safe "collective anchorage" as a counter position. The problem here is not the collective images of a given culture or of mankind, but the *specific* relatedness and cohesiveness of a group of individuals.
>
> (Moreno, 1960, pp. 116–117)

In one paragraph, Moreno identified a crucial deficiency in Jungian psychology that I also struggle with, as an analyst and group leader (Brooks, 2022). Jung did not apply the collective unconscious to the concrete collectivities, "*in which people* [also] *live,*" even though, as we have seen, his active imagination experiences were influenced by concrete socio-political events of his era. Jung's fidelity to the collective unconscious and the archetypes from which he theorized they emerged had the unfortunate effect of minimizing the influences that material environments have on our psychological development.[20] Graham, Lusijah, and I were prompted to write this book *because of this reality.* AIDS affected the psychological and social realities of human experience in our local community and world at large. Lusijah was the first beloved in my social network to viscerally feel the tragedy of AIDS and pulled me into the epicenter with her, along with Graham, Lucas, and others, who were already there. We had to adapt our treatment modalities and/or create new ones to creatively meet the demands of collective trauma described in Part II.

In my view, psychodrama group therapy is an activist arts-based methodology created to *socially* heal disenfranchised people within their communities (war refugees, sex workers, etc.), as described in Chapter 3. Moreno claimed that action techniques, such as psychodrama and sociodrama, were better equipped to explore the "co-conscious and co-unconscious" processes that were already activated in the experiences of group members (Moreno, 1960, pp. 113–117). While not excluding the viability of Jung's collective unconscious, Moreno highlighted a group's "natural function" to develop and share an unconscious life, through which its members could draw their "strength, knowledge and security" (Ibid.). Mutual aid approaches to group work, of any kind, draw on our natural function to cohere and mobilize towards mutually shared aims.

Tele, Mutuality Through Encounter, and Group Cohesion

Moreno formulated a concept he named "tele" that accounts for a group's capacity to cohere and form reciprocal relationships. Cohesion is essential to a group's capacity to authentically manifest mutual aid practices. Expressions of genuine mutual aid cannot be legislated. In psychodrama, we form, model, and nurture a culture that promotes mutual aid's possibility. John Olesen describes "tele" as a "mutual connection and communication of deep knowing that arises from a social encounter, and is the secret ingredient to forming diversified, group cohesion" (Olesen, Foreword of this book). Moreno (1960) determined he neither transference nor empathy were adequate explanations for the processes that foster cohesion that he regularly observed in psychodrama groups. His observations about tele and factors contributing to group cohesion were derived from numerous quantitative sociometric studies of group dynamics that he rigorously developed throughout his career (Moreno, 1953, 1960; Stephenson, 2014).[21]

Sociometric explorations reveal the often hidden structures, agenda, sub-groups, alliances, and belief systems that are operational in a group climate that hinder group cohesion, tele, and mutual aid.

Tele is a psychosocial factor that accounts for the mutuality of choices and for the increased rate of interaction between group members (Moreno, 1960, p. 18). Group action methods facilitate tele because they provide many opportunities for group members to encounter each other through role reversal, role playing, contact of bodies, confronting each other, sharing and loving, communicating, playing, seeing and perceiving, and participating in each other's psychodramas. Tele matures, in other words, through our multiple engagements with others while also deepening our authentic relationship with ourselves.

Tele, Active Imagination, and Archetypal Themes

In the spirit of cross-fertilization, we can say that Jung's method of active imagination, as noted in *The Red Book*, facilitated the development of his psychical tele and enhanced intrapsychic rapport with aspects of his personal and a collective psyche he had been ignoring. In active imagination, *we have to be open to receiving what psyche reveals. We don't imagine it.* The term active *imagination* is a misnomer because it implies the individual's imagination is a source of psyche (unconscious). *The unknown psyche is the source.* Psyche is enigmatic and generates traces through fantasies, dreams, images, visions, bodily sensations, symptoms, desire, affect, creative and destructive impulses, primary process, and speechlessness, to name a few. How we *engage with* the manifestation of psyche, however, *can be* imaginal, interpretative, creative, exploratory, performative, expressive, playful, thoughtful, art-making, and healing, thus generating new ways of understanding and being in the world.

When directing a psychodrama or leading a group process, I draw on active imagination as a vehicle for opening to the unconscious processes that are always present in the room that are verified and/or co-engaged with relationally. Let me be clear. I do not "receive from an outside all-knowing other" a universal truth of things. Psyche erupts, so to speak. Moreno might say that the sparks of co- and individual unconsciousness are rubbing against each other. What I "receive" needs to be metabolized and translated in relationship with others. I become my own methodologist, in other words an instrument of an unfolding process *with* group members that is always mysterious, uncertain, anxiety provoking, and sometimes transformative. A heuristic approach holds already formulated theories and practices *in balance with* a creative immersion in the work, organically creating new ways of being with what is happening *in situ*, as described in Chapter 6.

The psychodramatic stage provides a space for materializing psyche, in dialogue with one's depths, with each other, society, nature, and the "wisdom of centuries" (Rowland, 2023). I have come to think of archetypes as provisional universals or themes that arise synchronistically in a group or collective. Group members may be unaware of meaningful connections or patterns that underlie a group process until the psychophysiological continuum is activated and recognized. Collective themes have a universal shape and can be mapped accordingly (Lu & Yeoman, 2023). Turning points, moments of change, heightened polarities, impossible demands, crossroads situations, sudden reversals, and the revelation of synchronistic events may portend the appearance of an archetypal pattern or symbol. In Chapter 6, I discussed Connie's bleeding out as a psycho-activating, near-death event that held archetypal significance for the group. Connie's menstrual blood became a symbol of horror that constellated a truth about our shared precarity as human beings and the sacredness of life. When identified and interpreted, archetypes may become a basis for new consensual reality, in response to a dilemma posed, thus mobilizing the group towards a greater purpose beyond one's egoic desire. We may move, in other words, from personal concern to social responsiveness (Brooks, 2022).

Radical Love as an Archetype: Group Illustration

I will give you an illustration of how active imagination became a vector for a shared social concern from which tele was collectively nurtured and transformatively shared. In the Foreword of our book, John Olesen describes a psychodrama that I directed in the early AIDS era. I am circling to the beginning of our book to close the whole. This psychodrama centered around a young, dying protagonist's desire to have a lover, for the first time in his life, before he died. Death was imminent. John recalls: *"He might never know what it was to have a loving partner, and he was very sad."* As the protagonist arose, I joined him, as the psychodrama director. The simple action of physically joining him, standing beside him, and looking into his sad, full, eyes, opened me to a field between us. We were wading into the tidal flux between beings, what is known and unknown, mind and body, life and death, individual and collective, a *neptantla* space. My perceptual acuity became heightened, attentive, and expansive … taking in the whole and detail. We were opening to the dimension of ceremonial space where life and death are sacred. Not enough can be said about the feeling of what happens in ceremonial space, as its many dimensions are impossible to adequately describe. I opened to whatever would come, through him and the group. Perhaps we held hands. The group remained in the periphery of my awareness, alert, curious, agitated, engaged. His body was greatly weakened by the disease and worn down by a hopeless yearning for a lover. He knew it was, tragically, "too late," and yet there we were, on a threshold of his impossible desire and palpable grief. The poignancy of his yearning washed over me like a wave. Feeling the wave's crushing power, a thought emerged. Love is what he wants. Who among us doesn't want love? Perhaps he was conflating the role of having a lover with love itself. Love's impossibility was crushing his spirit. Material impossibility crashes into psychological possibility. Somewhere in between is where we stepped.

"Can we explore this?" I probably said. "Yes," he nodded. I turned towards the group, now opening to the collective psychic field that was *already there*, with us. Who will play the role of this man's lover? I asked. Hands slowly raised. Everybody was raising their hands. *"Everybody,"* as John describes it. How can we understand the loving animation that mobilized such a response except through love? It was time to materialize his impossible desire into a possible manifestation of love, in psychodramatic action. John refers to "the collective spell" we fell into as the protagonist received many kinds of loving from others who, like him, were also ill yet managed to physically maneuver the scenes, giving and receiving, one at a time, patiently, timelessly. We were all "lovers" now.

While disease could not be cured, the protagonist's suffering from *love loss* could be remedied. Love was the remedy. We cannot legislate love. His yearning tapped into a universal, the need for loving exchange. The participants in that room were all worn down from a collective loss of *Eros*, and treated as leper things because many were gay and carriers of a disease that was feared, misunderstood, and deadly. In this room, however, love became a remedy for collective exile, marginalization, disempowerment, and imminent death. Subversive love, love as activism, returning to the memory of wholeness through love, love as a socio-political, systemic, correction, love as an archetype, numinous love. The psychodrama transformed into a reparative ceremony for the group, where lost love is found again or newly experienced. Life's sacredness is momentarily restored.

Après Coup

A choral refrain throughout our book is this. Mutual aid–based groups and communities support the transformative possibility of *individual* and *group* development, where social change is possible in impossible situations. On a meta-level, we have seen how the development of a cohesive Quest community and eventual AIDS clinic in 1989 was a liberatory outcome of community individuation amidst broader, cross-cultural, social, and geo-political factors that sought to invisiblize the sacredness of life. In other words, the "synchronistic vertex" from which Quest emerged needs to be understood in the polarizing yet revolutionary context of AIDS activism (Lu & Yeoman, 2023).

In our view, the synchronistic vertex from which collective *Eros* may be restored in today's era is already happening in the revolutionary context of mutual aid activism. *The Healing Power of Community* is a call for care, beginning in our own house—the discipline of psychology. Group and community-based approaches to healing are a liberatory remedy for the systemic degradation of democratic values amidst broader socio/political factors that oppress the sacredness of all life. Mutual aid–influenced psychology is quietly gaining traction on the margins, emphasizing personal and group empowerment, social justice, and the centrality of mutual relationships. The possibilities are endless, calling us to creatively repair psychology's broken spirit, together.

Broadening the scope of psychology beyond the needs of the individual alone, and adapting mutual aid approaches to all levels of community engagement, can clarify and deepen the direction of psychology today. We hope that we have inspired our readers to push the boundaries of our field by placing mutual aid approaches at the very center of our clinical practice, advocacy, training, and research. The scope of psychology thus becomes elevated to the level of social change and political action. We believe there is a slow revolutionary turn towards community and group practice, whose embers we would like to enflame.

Notes

1 This portrayal of amplification is greatly simplified for the purposes of illustrating the method. The analysis I refer to was a long and complicated process, well beyond the perimeters of this chapter.

2 Jung was certainly influenced by the American psychologist William James, who had already differentiated logical thinking from associative thinking (Shamdasani, 2003).

3 Jung also engaged with figures that personify logos (mind), *Eros* (love), the "I," a fallen hero, Christ, demi-Gods, animals, reptiles, death and rebirth; these figures populate his visions.

4 Elsewhere, Jung wrote: "To really break with [a soul-deadening] tradition, one has to be willing to risk everything for it, to carry the experiment with [one's] own life through to the better end, and declare that [one's] life is not a continuation of the past, but a new beginning" (Jung, 1927/1970, para. 268).

5 The late philosopher Bernard Stiegler describes the sustaining effects of looming catastrophe in our era as contributing to "collective entropy." The forcefield of collective entropy suppresses our capacity to symbolize, imagine, and/or creatively think our way towards new "religious, spiritual, artistic, scientific, political movements, manners and styles, new institutions, social organizations, changes in education, in law, in forms of power and of course, changes in the very foundation of knowledge, whether this is conceptual knowledge, work-knowledge or life knowledge"(Stiegler, 2019, in Brooks, 2022, p. 46).

6 Jungian analyst Wolfgang Giegerich elaborates on this idea by postulating that the great questions, deep conflicts, and fundamental truths of any age come out of the effects of real, concrete events to which we are inured (Giegerich, 2004, p. 41).

7 Generally speaking, collectivist cultures emphasize the needs and goals of the group as a whole, such as in psychodrama, over the needs of the individual. Interconnectedness between people plays a critical role in each person's identity, in contrast with individualism where the personal needs of the individual take precedence. Within a mutual aid perspective, the individual and group contributes to the well-being (individuation) of each other.

8 The words of performance artist Laurie Anderson come to mind here in her performance piece entitled "World Without End": "*When my father died we put him in the ground, When my father died it was like a whole library had burned down.*" https://genius.com/Laurie-anderson-world-without-end-lyrics

9 Anzaldúa died before the actual *Red Book* was published but she had access to Jung's various descriptions of the process from which the method of active imagination would emerge described throughout his collected works. Anzaldúa's indebtedness to Jung and post-Jungian thought (James Hillman) is noted in many cited references throughout her works. Additionally, her master's thesis focused on "an archetypal approach" to literature where she referenced Jungian psychology (2009, p. 93).

10 Jungian analyst Wolfgang Giegerich describes the requirements of entering the "land of the self" that he likens it to experiencing a psychological death as we radically break from an old identity and sink into a process of forming another one (1999, p. 17).

11 Psychoanalyst Jacques Lacan builds on this idea by stating that we are not the agent of our own speech as much as it becomes through the act of speaking within the field of the other(s) (Lacan, 1999). We do not have our own language, in other words, because we are always embedded in the language and ideological discourses in our social and cultural networks from birth.

12 The capacity to care, or love ourselves, according to Jung depends on developing psychic rapport with our depths and repairing intra-psychical wounds that we are ignoring. From this basis, Jung makes a link with our capacity to care for others and "accept them with love," such as he did with the lifeless child found in the rubble heap of war (Jung, 2012, p. 344).

13 It is beyond the scope of this chapter to describe the seven steps of spiritual healing that Anzaldúa describes in her chapter entitled "Now let us shift…conocimiento… inner work, public acts" (2015, pp. 117–159).

14 Anzaldúa was a multi-disciplinarian and she attempted to write outside of official theoretical dogma. AnaLouise Keating identified her primary fields as creative writing, Queer theory, feminism, sexualities, gender, art, epistemology, literature, epistemology, spirituality, race, border culture, Raza (Chicano or Mexican-American identity, now Latinx), post-colonial studies, ethnic studies, and philosophy (Keating, Introduction, 2015, pp. 5–8). While Anzaldúa references Jung and James Hillman in particular, and Freud only occasionally, she does not include psychoanalysis or Jungian studies as a chief field of interest. Her extension of and application of Jung's method of active imagination, archetypal psychology, and theory of the transcendent function discussed in this chapter, however, highlight the degree to which their ontologies and methodologies overlap. See Fike (2018) for a lengthy discussion of Anzaldúa's appropriation of James Hillman's post-Jungian ideas.

15 Creative art therapies explosively emerged in the 20th century based on a variety of distinct orientations that include the integration of art forms as a therapy modality in group, individual, and community work (Malchiodi, 2018). With the advent of neurobiological developments in the last two decades, a shift towards integrating sensory-based therapeutic processes has become more popular because they provide access to the whole brain (both hemispheres) and to implicit and explicit memory (Siegel, 2012). Approaches that are body/whole brain and action oriented provide access to implicit memory, which is felt to be a key for wholistically treating psychological trauma (Van der Kolk, 2014, pp. 298–310).

16 I doubt that Anzaldúa would have considered her work to be Jungian arts-based research because she relied on *many* cultural, historical, and socio-political resources to decolonize personhood. She held the view that Western psychological concepts (Jung and mainstream psychology) were neither universally applicable nor superior to other ways of knowing derived from psycho/spiritual/socio/political/cultural contexts. Her work exemplifies how we might retain mainstream theories and practices that are applicable to non-Western human experience around the world. Thus, the very nature of psychology changes into an inclusive, multiplicitous, and global psychology.

17 In her first JABR mystery novel entitled *The Sacred Well Murders* (2022), Rowland reimagines a Celtic myth in a contemporary story featuring three female detectives who collaboratively solve the murder of a young woman while also highlighting climate change. Exploring the power of community to heal by making the unconscious conscious is a golden thread to her narrative. See also, Nikkel & Tamsen-Trent (2023).

18 See London Arts-based Research Centre – Transdisciplinary Conferences and Events: https://labrc.co.uk/

19 Cary Fink Baynes recalled Jung's description of the *Red Book* in 1923 as telling the story of the "battle between the world of reality and the world of the spirit" (Shamdasani, 2009, p. 213).

20 I use the following example of Jung's psychical obsession reported by Jungian analyst and child psychoanalyst Michael Fordham. Fordham recalls attempting to discuss child therapy at a dinner party with the Jungs. Of Jung, Fordham states: "He was starting on a monologue when Mrs. Jung intervened: 'You know very well that you are not interested in people, but [only] your theory of the collective unconscious'" (Fordham, 1975, pp. 102–113, in Brooks, 2019, pp. 130–131).

21 I strongly recommend the book entitled *Jung and Moreno* (2014), edited by Craig Stephenson and composed of essays written by Jungian scholars, analysts, psychotherapists, and psychodramatists.

References

Anderson, L. *World Without End.* https://genius.com/Laurie-anderson-world-without-end-lyrics. Accessed November 12, 2023.

Anzaldúa, B. (1981/2014). La Prieta. In C. Moraga & G. Anzaldúa (Eds.), *This Bridge Called My Back: Writings by Radical Women of Color*, pp. 198–209. Albany, NY: State University of New York Press.

Anzaldúa, G. (1987). *Borderlands/La Frontera: The New Mestiza.* San Francisco, CA: Aunt Lute Books.

Anzaldúa, G. (2000). *Interviews/Entrevistas/Gloria Anzaldúa.* New York: Routledge.

Anzaldúa, G. (2009). *The Gloria Anzaldúa Reader* (A. L. Keating, Ed.). Durham, NC: Duke University Press.

Anzaldúa, G. (2015). *Light in the Dark/Luz en lo Oscuro: Rewriting Identity, Spirituality, Reality* (A. L. Keating, Ed.). Durham, NC: Duke University.

Attinello, P. (2023). Splintered Afterlives: AIDS, Death and Beyond. In E. Broderson (Ed.), *Jungian Dimensions of the Mourning Process, Burial Rituals and Access to the Land of the Dead: Intimations of Immortality*, pp. 71–83. New York: Routledge.

Billig, M. (1997). The Dialogic Unconscious: Psychoanalysis, Discursive Psychology and the Nature of Repression. *British Journal of Social Psychology*, 36, 139–159.

Brooks, R. M. (2016). The International Transmission of the Catastrophic Effects of Real-world History Expressed in the Analytic Subject. In R. Naso & J. Mills (Eds.), *Ethics of Evil Psychoanalytic Explorations*, pp. 137–176. London: Karnac.

Brooks, R. M. (2019). A Critique of C. G. Jung's Theoretical basis for Selfhood. In J. Mills (Ed.), *Jung and Philosophy*, pp. 109–185. New York: Routledge.

Brooks, R. M. (2022). *Catastrophe, Psychoanalysis and Social Change.* New York: Routledge.

Brooks, R. M. (2023). C. G. Jung, Gloria Anzaldúa and Social Activism's Possibility. In L. Brodersen (Ed.), *Jungian Dimensions of the Mourning Process, Burial Rituals and Access to the Land of the Dead: Intimations of Immortality*, pp. 84–98. New York: Routledge.

Brown, L. & Strega, S. (Eds.) (2005). *Research as Resistance: Critical, Indigenous, & Anti-oppressive Approaches.* Toronto: Canadian Scholars' Press.

Carpani, S. (2021). Introduction – Andrew Samuels: Plurality, Politics and "the Individual." In S. Carpani (Ed.), *The Plural Turn in Jungian and Post-Jungian Studies: The Work of Andrew Samuels*, pp. 1–12. London: Routledge.

Chodorow, J. (Ed.). (1997). *Jung on Active Imagination.* Princeton, NJ: Princeton University Press.

Clarke, B. O. (2023). Synchronous Glitch: The Serious Play of Digital Matter. *Journal of Analytical Psychology*, 68(2), 443–447.

Crowley, K. (2011). *Feminism's New Age: Gender, Appropriation, and the Afterlife of Essentialism.* Buffalo, NY: State University of New York Press.

Fordham, M. (1975). Memories and Thoughts About C. G. Jung. *Journal of Analytical Psychology*, 20, 102–113.

Fike, M. A. (2018). Depth Psychology in Gloria Anzaldúa *Borderlands/La Frontera*: The New Mestiza. *Journal of Jungian Scholarly Studies*, 13. 52–70.

Frosh, S. & Baraitser, L. (2008). Psychoanalysis and Psychosocial Studies. *Psychoanalysis, Culture & Society*, 13, 346–365.

Giegerich, W. (2004). The End of Meaning and the Birth of Man. *Journal of Jungian Theory and Practice*, 6(1), 1–66.

Giegerich, W. (1999). *The Soul's Logical Life*. Frankfurt am Main: Peter Lang.

Hartman, T. (2021). *The Hidden History of American Healthcare: Why Sickness Bankrupts You and Makes Others Insanely Rich*. Oakland, CA: Berrett-Koehler Publishers.

Hinton, L. (2011). *Unus Mundus* – Transcendent Truth of Comforting Fiction – Overwhelm and the Search for Meaning in a Fragmented World. *Journal of Analytical Psychology*, 56(3), 375–380.

Hillman, J. & Shamdasani, S. (2013). *Lament of the Dead: Psychology after Jung's Red Book*. London: W. W. Norton.

Jung, C. G. (1912/1957/1967). *Symbols of Transformation*. CW 5. Princeton, NJ: Princeton University Press.

Jung, C. G. (1916/1957/1972). *The Transcendent Function*. CW 8. Princeton, NJ: Princeton University Press.

Jung, C. G. (1927/1970). *Women in Europe*. CW 10. Princeton, NJ: Princeton University Press.

Jung, C. G. (1928/1981). *On Psychoid Energy*. CW 8, Princeton, NJ: Princeton University Press.

Jung, C. G. (1935/1989). *The Tavistock Lectures*. CW 18. Princeton, NJ: Princeton University Press.

Jung, C. G. (1954/1975). *Psychological Commentary on "The Tibetan Book of the Great Liberation"*. CW 11. Princeton, NJ: Princeton University Press.

Jung, C. G. (1971). *Schiller's Ideas on the Type Problem*. CW 6. Princeton, NJ: Princeton University Press.

Jung, C. G. (1998). *Nietzsche's Zarathustra: Notes of the Seminar Given in 1934–1937* (J. Jarrett, Ed.). London: Routledge.

Jung, C. G. (2009). *The Red Book: Liber Novus* (S. Shamdasani, Ed.; M. Kyburz, J. Peck, & S. Shamdasani, Trans.). New York and London: W. W. Norton.

Jung, C. G. (2012). *The Red Book, Liber Novus. A Reader's Edition.* (S. Shamdasani, Trans.). New York and London: W. W. Norton.

Keating, A. (2015). *Editor's Introduction*. In G. Anzaldúa, *Light in the Dark/Luz en lo Oscuro: Rewriting Identity, Spirituality, Reality*, pp. ix–xxxviii. Durham, NC and London: Duke University Press.

Lacan, J. (1999). *The Seminar of Jacques Lacan: On Feminine Sexuality, the Limits of Love and Knowledge* (J. A. Miller, Ed.). New York: W.W. Norton and Company.

Lacan, J. (2014). *Anxiety: The Seminar of Jacques Lacan: Book X* (J. A. Miller, Ed.; A. R. Price, Trans.). Cambridge: Polity Books.

Lu, K. & Yeoman, A. (2023). The Future of Jungian Psycho-Social Studies: Akira, Greta Thunberg and Archetypal Thematic Analysis (ATA). *International Journal of Jungian Studies*.

Lu, K. (2020). Racial Hybridity: Jungian and Post Jungian Perspectives. *International Journal of Jungian Studies*, 12, 11–40.

Malchiodi, C. A. (2018) Creative Arts Therapies and Arts-Based Research. In P. Leavy (Ed.), *Handbook of Arts-Based Research*, pp. 68–87. New York: Guilford Press.

Moreno, J. L. (1953). *Who Shall Survive? Foundations of Sociometry, Group Psychology and Sociodrama*. Beacon, NY: Beacon House Inc.

Moreno, J. L. (1960). Sociometric Base of Group Psychotherapy. In J. L. Moreno, H. H. Jennings, J. H. Criswell, L. Katz, R. R. Blake, J. S. Mouton, M. E. Bonney, M. L. Northway, C. P. Loomis, C. Proctor, R. Tagiuri, & J. Nehnevajsa (Eds.), *The Sociometry Reader*, pp. 113–117. Glencoe, IL: The Free Press.

Moreno, J. L. (1971). *The Words of the Father*. Beacon, NY: Beacon House.

Musso, V. C. (2023). The Day of the Dead in Los Angeles as Numinosum: How Honoring the Dead Reconnects Mexican Americans to their Aztec-Mexica Ancestral Roots. In E. Brodersen (Ed.), *Jungian Dimensions of the Mourning Process, Burial Rituals and Access to the Land of the Dead: Intimations of Immortality*, pp. 17–29. New York and London: Routledge.

Nikkel, D. & Tamsen-Trent, H. (2023). *The Sacred Well Murders* (2022). Jungian Arts-Based Research (JABR) in Action. *Journal of Analytical Psychology, 68*(2), 440–442.

Pearse, H. (1983). Brother, Can You Spare a Paradigm? The Theory beneath the Practice. *Studies in Art Education, 24*(3), 158–163.

Pitts, A. J. (2021). *Nos/Ostras: Gloria E. Anzaldúa, Multiplicitous Agency, and Resistance.* Albany, NY: Sunny Press.

Rolling, J. H. (2013). *Arts-Based Research Primer.* New York: Peter Lang.

Rolling, J. H. (2018). Arts-Based Research in Education. In P. Leavy (Ed.), *Handbook of Arts-based Research*, pp. 493–510. New York: Guilford Press.

Rowland, S. (2023). Jungian Arts-Based Research (JABR): What It Is, Why Do It, and How. *Journal of Analytical Psychology, 68*(2), 436–439.

Rowland, S. (2022), *The Sacred Well Murders*. Asheville, NC: Chiron Publications.

Rowland, S. & Weishaus, J. (2021). *Jungian Arts-based Research and the Nuclear Enchantment of New Mexico.* New York: Routledge.

Ruiz, E. R. (2020). Between Hermeneutic Violence and Alphabets of Survival. In A. J. Pitts, M. Ortega, & J. Medina (Eds.), *Theories of Flesh, Latinx and Latin American Feminisms, Transformation, and Resistance*, pp. 204–219. New York: Oxford University Press.

Saban, M. (2020). Simondon and Jung: Rethinking Individuation. In C. McMillian, R. Main, & D. Henderson (Eds.), *Holism: Possibilities and Problems*, pp. 91–97. London and New York: Routledge.

Saban, M. (2019). *"Two Souls Alas": Jung's Two Personalities and the Making of Analytical Psychology.* Asheville, NC: Chiron Publications.

Samuels, A. (2015). Global Politics, American Hegemony and Vulnerability and Jungian Psychosocial Studies: Why There Are No Winners in the Battle Between Trickster Pedro Urdemales and the Gringos. *International Journal of Jungian Studies, 7*(3), 227–241.

Shamdasani, S. (2003). *Jung and the Making of Modern Psychology: A Dream of a Science.* Cambridge: Cambridge University Press.

Shamdasani, S. (Ed.) (2009). Introduction. In M. Kyburtz, J. Peck, & S. Shamdasani (Trans.), *The Red Book: A Reader's Edition*, pp. 1–113. New York: W. W. Norton.

Siegel, D. (2012). *The Developing Mind: How Relationships and the Brain Intersect to Shape Who We Are.* New York: Guilford Press.

Springgay, S. (2002). Arts-Based Research as an Uncertain Text. *The Alberta Journal of Educational Research, 48*(3), 1–30.

Stephenson, C. E. (2014). *Jung and Moreno: Essays on the Theatre of Human Nature.* New York and London: Routledge.

Stiegler, B. (2019). *The Age of Disruption: Technology and Madness in Computational Capitalism* (D. Ross, Trans.). Medford, MA: Polity Books.

Swan-Foster, N. (2018). *Jungian Art Therapy: A Guide to Dreams, Images, and Analytical Psychology.* New York and London: Routledge.

Van der Kolk, B. (2014). *The Body Keeps the Score.* New York: Viking.

Watkins, M. & Shulman, H. (2008). *Toward Psychologies of Liberation.* New York: Palgrave Macmillan.

Wetherell, M. (2003). Paranoia, Ambivalence and Discursive Practices: Concepts of Position and Positioning in Psychoanalysis and Discursive Psychology. In R. Harré & F. Moghaddam (Eds.), *The Self and Others: Positioning Individuals and Groups in Personal, Political and Cultural Contexts*, pp. 99–120. New York: Praeger/Greenwood Publishers.

Index

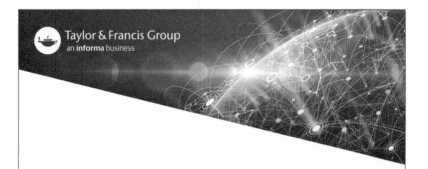